The God Gap

A Mother's Miraculous Journey to Find
Healing for Her Son's Acquired Brain Injury

———

Kim Russell, M.Ed.

The God Gap

A Mother's Miraculous Journey to Find Healing for Her Son's Acquired Brain Injury

Cover design by:

SpeakTruth Media Group LLC

Published by:

SpeakTruth Media Group LLC

Back Cover Photo:

Grace Photography by Jill Ingram Sellers

gracephotographybyjill@gmail.com

For information about special discounts available for bulk purchases, sales promotions, fundraising, and educational needs, contact by email: SpeakTruth Media Group LLC at order@speaktruthmedia.com.

ISBN: 979-8-9857296-0-3 *(pb)*

Printed in the USA

DEDICATION

To my mom, my greatest supporter, she was always there during every challenge. When she went to heaven, I often felt like an orphan. I thought I couldn't do life without her. Now I realize that it was God all along Who led me through every difficulty, and for that, I'm eternally grateful.

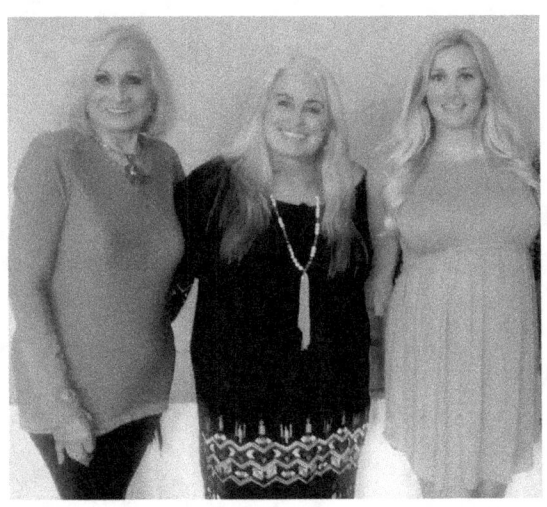

CONTENTS

TESTIMONIALS

I love Kim's energy and passion to serve others. She is a true servant leader with a desire to make the world a better place.

— Julie Toth

I'm extremely blessed to know Kim Russell as a business partner and friend. She has a huge heart for loving others, seeing the good in everyone, and always believing the best. Kim has a calming presence, which perfectly fits her education and equine therapy work. Her wisdom about life, relationships, love, and science combines effortlessly, making her an incredible friend and mentor. Above all else, her passion and love as a mother is felt in every conversation. Nothing can get in her way of helping someone she loves, and her journey with Mitchell is a true testament to her determination to not only get her son back but to help other families needing the same. In my opinion, Kim is an *angel* on earth.

— Susann Crowell

I met Kim Russell on August 11, 2011, at the Tasting Room in Uptown Park. We didn't talk much that day, but the date became significant for several reasons, but our paths became profoundly connected. Over the years, we traveled many miles together literally and figuratively, and I am proud to call her friend. One thing I know for sure, Kim is meant to change lives with her special gifts and knowledge.

When we met, she was working to save her equine therapy facility; Morning Glory Ranch, which catered to children with special needs, autism, and PTSD. While her background as an educational leader set the stage for her unique insight into how the brain and body "function," her biology acumen and 20 years of graduate research into cell chemistry would play an important role in her life, and ultimately through Mitchell's journey, this book.

Mitchell and my daughter are the same age and friends, both traveled with us on all sorts of adventures, so when his behavior changed, there was no denying that something serious was unfolding. Her painful recognition of her fears and feelings of inadequacy while handling each trauma produce both intrinsic and practical lessons for us all. The last few years have been her dedicated quest to find a formula for healing her son. The trials and failed attempts were not in vain; she gives hope and insights to others by sharing their journey.

In her book, The God Gap, you will learn more about how the body functions and heals in tiny increments, often slower than we desire.

Shining through it all, is a mother's heart of fierce love. I hope that her heartbreaks and joy will also bring you comfort on your journey.

— Carla Hill

ACKNOWLEDGMENTS

Let me take a moment to acknowledge the people who have inspired and believed in me along the way. Each of you gave me the strength to stay the course and fight in faith every day.

To my son Mitchell inspires me along with many other children with acquired brain injuries. He is a warrior determined to stay as loving and kind as he has always been. His fight to be whole will always give me the inspiration I need to continue my work as a researcher.

To my husband, who stood beside us, spent 15 years raising Mitchell as a part of his life and continues today to be there for us is a source of tremendous strength to me. A part of me chases things to prove people wrong, and I know that's not the Jesus way. David, I have put you through a lot, but I want you to know that I love you, and I'm grateful for you every day.

To my Morning Glory Ranch family—clients, donors, staff, and volunteers—who all prayed for us daily. Along with Mitchell and my family, you helped me stay focused on Jesus, which helped me discover the *God Gap*. And, to our horses, I thank God for His creation of such magnificent animals that have an empathetic sense and bring healing to those who need it most.

To my publisher Charlana Kelly and SpeakTruth Media, without the Holy Spirit bringing her to me at the perfect time, this book would have never been written. She encouraged and prayed with me, sharing the instruction I needed. I am a thinker and a dreamer who spends most of her life in her imagination. Charlana showed me that I could do the impossible; write a book and inspire the world.

And finally, to all the people and *angels*, I needed to open my eyes.

FOREWORD

Mitchell Smith is a child in a man's body.

I came into his life after he was arrested on Christmas day of 2017. On that day, Mitchell and his family went to Santa's Wonderland – a Christmas light tour and recreation area where millions of decorative lights complement seasonal activities. The experience at Santa's Wonderland can be overwhelming – even to a neurotypical person.

Mitchell was not a neurotypical person. Without provocation, Mitchell assaulted a woman and was arrested. He was held in the Brazos County Jail from that date until early March, when he was found incompetent to stand trial, and his criminal charge was dismissed. Simultaneous with that dismissal, I assisted in creating a temporary guardianship.

Additional evaluations and investigations revealed acquired brain injuries (ABIs) resulting from numerous concussions sustained by Mitchell while playing youth and high school football.

These ABIs were exacerbated by Mitchell's use of K2 – a

synthetic cannabinoid containing mind-altering substances marketed and intended to produce the same effect as illegal drugs. K2 use and the ABIs created a synergistic effect. As a result, Mitchell's ability to care for himself and function in society deteriorated over months.

In May of 2018, Mitchell was named as a permanent ward when Brazos County Court at Law #1 found that he was incapacitated, which included an inability to care for himself, manage his property, operate a motor vehicle, make personal decisions regarding his residence, or vote in a public election. By order of the Court, Mitchell's mother, Kim Russell, was appointed his legal guardian. This order required Kim to exercise all the powers, rights, and duties given to a Guardian in the Texas Estates Code. This guardianship essentially obligated Kim to care for her twenty-one-year-old son as she did when he was a child.

The powers specifically included, but are not limited to were

The right to have physical possession of the Ward and to arrange for Mitchell's food and housing needs,

The power to arrange for any medical, psychological, and dental tests, evaluations, and care, disclosing confidential records as necessary

The power to apply for and secure governmental services and an identification care for Mitchell, and

The power to execute all documents necessary to facilitate employment.

Unlike many similarly situated wards, Mitchell was lucky that he had a mother dedicated to improving her son's quality of life who would not take no for an answer. Kim was determined to see her son heal. She sacrificed a career and neglected other family obligations to focus on Mitchell's condition by her own admission. She sought out scientific resources to aid in Mitchell's recovery.

She used her professional contacts and life experiences to aid Mitchell in regaining his cognitive abilities. She relied on trusted professionals in the medical, therapeutic, and legal world to assist her when she encountered situations beyond her ability.

When I contemplate the relationship between Mitchell and

Kim, I can't help but reflect on the biblical role of a mother articulated in Proverbs chapter 31 verses 25-28:

25 She is clothed with strength and dignity,

and she laughs without fear of the future.

26 When she speaks, her words are wise,

and she gives instructions with kindness.

27 She carefully watches everything in her household

and suffers nothing from laziness.

28 Her children stand and bless her.

Verses that become even more meaningful when I think of Kim's love and dedication to her son. With so many uncertainties in our world, it is easy to be driven by fear and worry rather than faith. Kim's moral (as a mother) and legal responsibility (as a guardian) for the safety of Mitchell could have consumed her to the point that she became too scared to take chances and too worried about what the future might hold.

It is typical for parents to be anxious about what the future holds for their children. Being afraid of the unknown and feeling worried is normal; those feelings do not drive a virtuous mother. According to the words from Proverbs 31, God has given Kim the ability to "laugh at the days to come."

Kim Russell takes comfort that God can give a kind of peace that surpasses all understanding. She faces the future with boldness and confidence, knowing that God is beside her through it all – filling the God Gap.

Open this book, read it, and pray on its message. Inspiration will follow.

— Mark Maltsberger

INTRODUCTION

Ours is an incredible story. It is not all good incredible. Some of it is exceptionally incredible. However, some of it is awful, shocking, shameful, and embarrassing. But all of it is real. And our story is an offering to parents who have similar stories of their own. For the last six years, the journey we have been on has held disappointment, discouragement, frustrations, fear, guilt, and shame. But our journey does not end there, thank God. It ends with discovery, recovery, reconciliation, and restoration, with wild hope and immutable faith in a loving God who brought us through the valley of the shadow of death!

Wild hope! A hope that did not come easily but was born out of struggles that completely overwhelmed us in a situation where we did everything we knew to do and still didn't have the answers we ultimately needed. We sought experts, implemented every plan and possibility. There were many trials and errors, while we discovered and learned as we went. In our pursuit, we were forced to watch our beloved son tossed about like a ragdoll with dysfunction brought on by injuries that seemed to defy an explanation until our research offered one. Like buried treasured, we sifted through mounds of research, ideas, and treatments, relevant and not until we found answers in the light that only God could reveal to us! Our successes were beyond diligent human effort. In the end, success came from what can only be described as an empty place where we had nothing left to offer. BUT GOD! He provided what we were glaringly lacking and could not fathom. All while responding with love, patience, mercy, forgiveness, and healing, both physical and emotional.

As I began putting this book together, I experienced an unmanageable gamut of emotions: excitement, confusion, fear, and eventually profound courage. Knowing that I would lay open our lives for the scrutiny of others left me reeling with doubt and questions of what others might think of us. Would anyone be able to relate to our experiences and pain, then ultimately our love and joy? Is there a purpose for documenting this emotional saga, or would others be better served with the science and facts behind what we learned? I agonized through self-evaluation and the honest admissions required to admit where I was in my relationship with my son, husband, and God. It was the most challenging lesson I ever had to learn. It was also the most life-changing, rewarding, and satisfying time of my entire life.

I learned that to release guilt, shame, and remorse; I had to face the facts head-on with raw honesty. I had to acknowledge the truths about my life, good, bad, or ugly, and repent. I surrendered my hold on my life, ideas, and way of doing things, and I put all my trust in God. To acknowledge it was challenging to let go completely is a mammoth understatement. However, I gave control to God. It was a massive shift to put my hope in the unseen, a place that I could not touch nor see. I call this place the God Gap. And I have found that surrendering everything and everyone, including myself, to live in the God Gap has forever changed me! I found the faith, knowledge, and courage to leave behind the darkness that had flooded my soul for so long. Each day is a gift. Now I wake up and thank Jesus for what I have and the mission He has given me to serve Him, my family, and others with the best ability He has given me.

As you follow our story, I hope you can benefit from seeing the knowledge we gained on the difficult path we took to where God was the only answer. And I hope you can recognize the place of honest surrender in your own life as you allow the love of God to change and inspire you as well.

— Chapter 1 —

RETRACING DESTINY

It's been said that our lives are predestined. As I reflected on my life to write this book, I was amazed as I retraced God's path for me. My mom always reminded me that when I was in kindergarten, I told everyone I wanted to be a brain surgeon when we were asked what we wanted to be when we grew up. In hindsight, it kind of came true. You decide.

I spent 25 years in public education, most of that coaching and teaching biology, biochemistry, and special education. I was a club mentor, which I loved. Ultimately, I became an administrator of a Title I school in 1999, where I realized children with behavioral issues need to be educated differently than what we were delivering. So, I started putting together the knowledge and experience I had gleaned from years of preparation. As a result, I began approaching kids and their learning differently.

Many kids came to school carrying emotional baggage that they were too immature to know how to deal with it. I grew up with horses and owned horses at that time. I decided to focus on the kids who were frequently in my office for discipline issues. I affectionately called them the frequent flyers and began to take them to my Ranch to interact with the horses. It was magical to watch what the horses were doing to instill hope and give these kids a foundation for communication. What seemed to be missing most in their lives was unconditional love and a place where they could express themselves in an emotionally safe environment.

I remember James, a 13-year-old student living with his grandmother in extreme poverty. Super quiet and emotionally fragile, James trusted no one. He had kind eyes behind his hurt, spending most of his time in my office at school, mainly for not following directions. The more I got to know and listen to James, the more I understood he needed someone to be proud of him. He also needed someone to hug him until those walls came down, leaving him in tears. James was one of the first students who went to the Ranch. Often, I found him with the horses in the small pasture talking away, speaking more words than I had ever heard him say. By the end of that school year, James was riding and, at one point, trusted the horse enough to stand on its back! James found his dreams and passions that year. He became one of our first peer instructors for our first student with autism.

We learned that experiential education was what these kids needed. Since I could monitor their behavioral changes, we noted what was and wasn't working. I began writing a curriculum based on how these horses instilled hope and confidence in the students, helping them see their value and possibilities for the future. I believed their interaction with the horses would make the most significant impact on their lives. I watched as these kids began to thrive and even become more giving.

Seeing the potential outcomes for these children, I attended

Rice University to learn about non-profit leadership. I wanted to

turn what I was doing with these kids into a foundation that would

focus primarily on
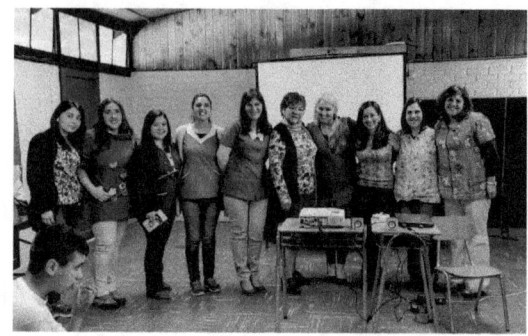
helping disadvantaged

children. In June 1999,

Morning Glory Ranch

(MGR) was born. Initially, our focus was to provide horse therapy

for children with behavioral concerns. The program we offered

quickly expanded to include special needs children, mostly those

with acquired brain injuries (ABI). Soon afterward, we began

serving kids with autism, Down syndrome, severe behavioral

disorders, attention-deficient / hyperactive disorder (ADHD), and

a few with developmental delays. You should have seen the looks

of pride on the faces of our behavioral students as they taught and

shared what they learned about the horses and the Ranch with the

special needs kids. We were pretty proud to see this ourselves and

were thrilled as we began to see these children succeed in their academic classes as well. What we were doing was working!

Morning Glory Ranch grew by leaps and bounds, especially when we started seeing so much progress with Autistic children. Much of that success was in fundamental food changes by simply adding more fruits and vegetables. Factor in their experiences with other students, other instructors, their horses, and the entire ranch atmosphere; we created an environment that changed and improved lives.

In the Summer of 2006, we moved the Ranch from Wharton to Waller, Texas, and began operating on 25 acres with a small barn. I had taken a job in special education at a junior high school and quickly noticed that the education system was becoming political. When I was asked to make decisions that I knew were not suitable for kids, I knew it was time to leave. My daughter Kaydee was headed to Texas A&M University to play softball, and I wanted to be there for her. We had created an educational program successfully working at the Ranch, and I could easily see the areas where our program could grow. The public system was not open to providing the extracurricular opportunities I could provide to the kids, so in May 2010, I walked away.

I experienced huge fear while making that decision! Education had been my life, yet I left that successful twenty-five-year career. Suddenly I had no job, no income, two kids in college, one still in high school, and an eleven-year-old charity doing amazing things for children and families. Add to this the fact that our country was amid a substantial economic turndown in 2010, which meant an awful economy, no non-profit dollars, or donor money. Charities such as ours exist through donations. Operating becomes extremely difficult when people have no money to give or no job to generate extra income. I had become a professional beggar over the eleven years the Ranch was active. I was very good at sharing about our program, the success the kids were experiencing, and getting lots of donations to support our organization. Things were quite different now.

Part of me was terrified as I adjusted to this new place, yet part of me was at peace. I wasn't working, had no personal funds, and now no non-profit dollars coming in. It was a moment that would require a massive pivot in my life. I had major decisions to make. Do I play it safe? Play it small? Downsize and cut things out? Or do I keep dreaming big and pushing forward with faith? As you may guess, I'm not a quitter, but this was overwhelming. When obstacles arise and big changes charge up against you, what do you do? What do you do when God says, "You've got to stop. That's it."?

My response? I sat down in my pasture and had a conversation with fifteen horses. Those horses were saying, "Don't sell me, mom. Don't sell me." It was a tremendous burden to decide that, knowing it would impact my own kids' lives plus the lives of a hundred families depending on therapy every week. There were other considerations with our staff, volunteers, and donors. It was undoubtedly the biggest decision of my life, and it would require greater faith than I ever had before.

I threw up my arms and said the most powerful and heartfelt prayer I'd ever said in my life. I implored God, "Please don't send me back to public school; please put me where I need to be." It was simple and real. At that moment, I needed His help before going any further.

GOD PUT ME WHERE I NEEDED TO BE

For decades I have been an avid researcher, reading scientific papers almost daily and studying the invisible world of biochemistry. It is what drives me, sends my creativity reeling, and motivates me to find a solution that can help my families at the Ranch. So, I did what I knew to do. I packed up and headed for Utah to attend a meeting about plant extracts beneficial for autistic children. I got upgraded to first-class on the plane, which had never happened before, and I never wanted to waste the money to purchase it for myself. I felt honored to be moved up and was overwhelmed with gratitude as I enjoyed my blessing. The man that sat beside me was also upgraded, then, God winked.

Dr. Bill was in a clinical trial using plant extracts that align with the research I have been doing. As soon as I heard that, I started trembling. We chatted for three hours, and I explained what we had been doing at Morning Glory Ranch and the successes we were experiencing. He knew and understood what we were doing and was excited about it. Near the end of the flight, I asked him, "Where are you from?" and when he answered, "Waller, Texas," I was stunned! "That is where our charity is!" Then Dr. Bill adds, "Really? We were just looking for a charity to support!" It was as if God met me at 35,000 feet and said, "Alright, it's time for you to listen up. Here is your path."

After this "chance" encounter, all our endeavors took a miraculous turn. Dr. Bill and his wife Julie introduced me to innovative products that already had scientific substantiation by a world-renown company. As a charity founder, I was often approached by companies that wanted to sell me their products, but this was different. And it was wonderful! And I knew this was Divine intervention. I had done years of research, worked with many families of children with autism, and conferred with doctors, but their contributions were nothing like this. What was unfolding was absolutely ingenious and way outside the box of mainstream wellness. We were about to tap the cellular source of life!

As a result, my husband David and I partnered with the most prominent genetic anti-aging research and development company globally. We set our course toward learning about cellular nourishment healing. It was biochemistry and wellness at its most complex yet simple concept. We had world-class testing and measurement capabilities at our disposal that allowed us to make individual adjustments. It was a true game-changer because it provided us a way to empower families to know if what they were doing for their child every day was working. That's huge—no more guessing.

Families of children with special needs, any particular need like anxiety, depression, even schizophrenia, psychosis, Down syndrome, anything, they're all looking for hope. They're looking for something that can help them in their day-to-day life. And this was it! Nourishing these children at the cellular level was the missing piece for these families. We brought in the technology and began the supplementation, then were able to measure their level of antioxidant cell protection. We began measuring all the children in the program, their families, staff, donors, the entire community. And we were doing this with a global database and Nobel Prize-winning technology. What we were offering was world-class.

However, my belief and excitement were not enough. Half our clients left because they couldn't wrap their heads around what we were doing, which was a blow to the charity. I was devasted and began to second guess myself. Funding for a charity is dependent on the number of participants. We were in trouble once again. Julie, Dr. Bill's wife, sat me down and asked point-blank how much money we needed to continue. Ten thousand dollars a month! It was a lot. But she had been with our company for a decade and knew what was possible. I followed everything she and Dr. Bill said and stayed close to them as mentors. I wholeheartedly felt what we had our hands on was significant. I was not giving up. I was going to keep going until we won! I felt God led me there for a reason, and I was determined to take it to the finish line. I knew I could save the charity; I just didn't know how to do it. Yet!

We began to network. Many people, doctors, and therapy centers around the country became involved, even a few in other countries. For four years, we focused on collecting the data results from cellular nourishment. Lots of it. We noticed considerable changes in the functions of the kids in the program. I then designed a research protocol where we could measure that function over time and included not only children with autism but also those with different levels of acquired brain injuries (ABI). The beauty of this was that we had a concrete measurement that was non-invasive and did not require parents to drag their kid to a doctor for regular blood work and all the trauma that goes with that. God continued to give me a vision. I knew this was what I wanted to do; empower families and watch these moms have a way to make a difference in their kids' lives. And so, we did that. In the process, we were able to generate funds for the charity. I did not see that coming at all! It was God's provision because, in six years, we generated over a million dollars!

The Morning Glory Ranch name and brand, what we were doing, our mission and vision for supporting these children were spreading—and spreading like wildfire! Many folks said, "What are you doing? Will it help my child?" And my answer was, "Every child is the study of 'one.' But I can tell you right now, 100% of the kids in the study have had an increase in function at some level." It was great news to parents! At this time in America, prevention wellness was NOT a thing. Have an issue? Pop a pill to fix it. That was the norm—immediate gratification with little concern for long-term improvement. We were doing something important, innovative, and life-changing!

The provision came to Morning Glory Ranch in extraordinary ways. We built a 45,000 square foot roof over the equestrian center in one YEAR. Our dream became a reality as the Ranch became an all-inclusive acquired brain injury facility. We were serving lots of children, families, and communities. There was so much energy, love, and power in this covered arena and plenty of space for the kids to be safe, have fun, and grow in a peaceful, happy state. And parents were able to take a breather from the minute-to-minute stress of parenting a challenging child with acquired brain injury.

We experienced astonishing success, and I was on a mission to teach everything we discovered. In four and a half years, I presented our information and shared our successes in eleven countries. It was a whirlwind as I traveled extensively, but I loved every minute of this incredible time! Through it all, I felt God was indeed leading us to measure nutritional antioxidant absorption

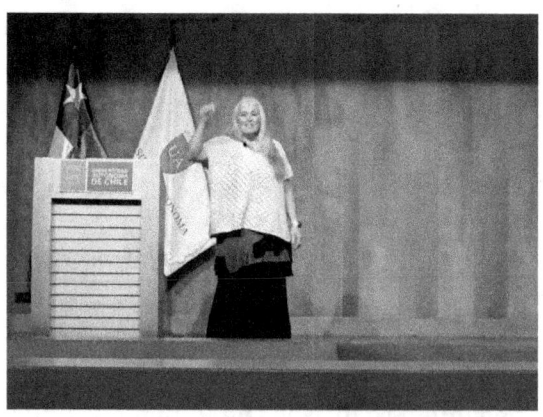

for every kid in the world! We could make it happen! I felt like I was on top of the world, and we were about to conquer it!

In November of 2016, the University of Autonoma in Santiago in Chile was our last stop. I was nervous because everything had to be translated into Spanish. What should have taken about 45 minutes expanded to nearly three hours as I had to pause and wait for the translator. I was relieved to have this last presentation completed and was glad to be heading home. I met some fantastic folks there who continue to be part of my life. After finishing, I felt a great sense of self-satisfaction.

Then, abruptly, my life as I had known it completely crashed around my feet.

— Chapter 2 —

THE CALL I NEVER IMAGINED

My twenty-year-old son Mitchell was catatonic, which meant that he could not eat, drink, or handle bodily functions on his own. He could barely walk, even with maximum assistance. I learned that he had what was termed primal brain shutdown. Fear struck my heart; I was terrified. I faced a deluge of emotions I had never experienced. I had so many questions, the biggest: Why did God do this? And, what is happening with my son?

Here is where my story gets hard.

Mitchell is the youngest of my three children. Most of

Mitchell's childhood is a blur to me. I tried to remember the good things from when he was little, but sadly, not many memories of good things popped up. Not because he didn't have them, but because I was not in sync with him at the time. I spent nearly two decades focused on my career, charity, travels, and teaching, basically determined to help other children. It is excruciating for me to admit how disconnected I was from Mitchell during his childhood and school years.

Mitchell was a happy baby. During those years, he was my superman, in his cape, running across the roof of our house. He was my little artist and went everywhere with his sister Kaydee and me, drawing in the car while we were flying down the road. Nothing deterred his focus. Often, he would take that art and sell it at the ballpark earning money to spend at the concession stand. He was an start up entrepreneur.

Once, at age five, he hopped on a horse, took off across the corn field, and dispatched me to scramble after him. I saddled up and chased him in a trail of dust. Afterward, all my little freedom-seeker could say was, "I didn't fall off, Mom!" while laughing hysterically. It's funnier to me now than it was then.

Always kind-hearted, Mitchell was my giver. He jumped in to help our special needs children when they arrived then stayed with them during their lessons on the horses. He was quick to keep others safe, and his demeanor was consistently loving.

One of my biggest regrets was that I failed to make a strong connection with him during his teen years. I was gone a lot, too much, I realize in retrospect. I allowed other people to fulfilled Mitchell's needs. It hurts me deeply now to admit that I sometimes felt resentful that I had to take care of him when he was little. I was doing important work in my eyes and was put off by my own child's demands on me. His brother and sister were 7 and 5 years older than Mitchell. They were much more self-sufficient by then. Today, I wish I could just go back and do this part all over again.

After the shutdown and all the trials, work, and pain they brought, I had lots of time to reflect on what led to that moment in November 2016. At times, acknowledging the truth about where I was in relationship with my family has been overwhelming. Still, my willingness to process the events and fallout allowed me to dig deep into who I am as a mother, a wife, and a person. It has not been easy. It has been heart-wrenching. I'm not sure I have an appropriate adjective to describe the pit of despair I have navigated. But I wish it on no one.

Hindsight is always 20/20. Anguish, resentment, and many tears have brought me to these revelations. Here's the good news though, I have come through it all!! As you face difficulties in your life, be assured, there is a way out. Help is there for you. God was faithful to me year after year before I could even acknowledge that He was there. He is there for you too. Hang in there. My story continues.

I came out of a wretched abusive marriage when Mitchell was four. When he was ten, David moved in with us, and we married a year later. The kids and I had been a family of four but things were changing, and like any other blended family, there were challenges. Mitchell wanted to sleep in our room, which was not appropriate.

David, of course, didn't take too kindly to it. David resented Mitchell, and because I didn't know how to handle this from a right perspective at that time, his resentment increased over the years. I was so torn. I wanted to honor my husband, but I wanted to be there for Mitchell. Knowing what I know now, I would have made a different choice if I had a chance to do it over. Through my traveling years, the strain between them escalated.

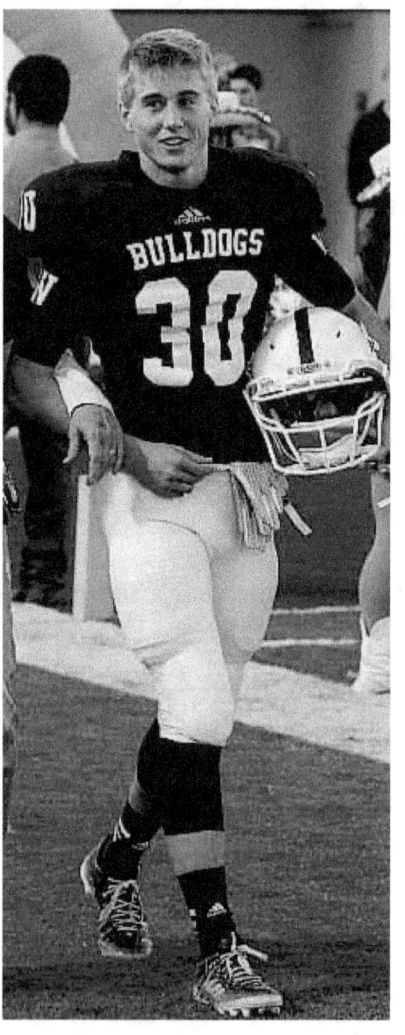

Mitchell was a natural athlete. He began playing Pee Wee football around age ten, like his brother and sister. There were 12 boys from the pee wee days that stayed friends and played football together through high school graduation, the beauty of a small town. I remember that

Mitchell's uniform was way too big, which necessitated us buying pants for him. We also bought him the best helmet money could buy at the time, and I do not recall him ever sustaining a football injury. The game was huge part of his life. In Mitchell's teenage years, he had great friends around mostly football players and lots of girls. He was an above-average student and a country boy with a big Dodge truck, blond hair, and a beautiful girlfriend. He was well-liked by everyone and seldom alone.

Mitchell and his brother Michael often played the Madden Football video games together and attended Michael's varsity football games. Mitchell looked up to his brother, and they spent a lot of time together. When Michael went out with friends, Mitchell was included, and if the older boys were drinking, Mitchell became the driver. At twelve! I always wondered how he learned to drive so well. They told me years later. Then, sadly, after Michael left for college, they hardly ever saw each other.

In seventh grade, Mitchell Started having some issues in a couple of classes at school. He had problems in Spanish, but I was like, hey, I get that. I can't speak Spanish either. But it was more like he didn't want to try, which was odd for him. And then he started struggling in his English class, mainly because he didn't want to write anything. I was super busy and did not pay attention to it. I did not view his new behaviors and attitudes as a red flag, so I didn't get him the needed help. I saw him as a typical boy in puberty. I totally missed it.

Mitchell's sister Kaydee was a second mama to him. She watched out for him and spent a lot of time with him. She taught him how to ride his bike and took him shopping. He always looked sharp thanks to 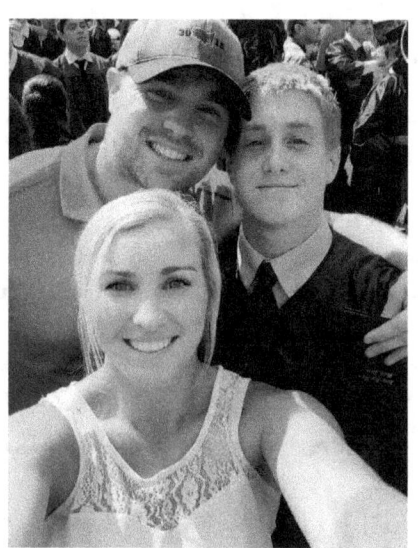 her and was almost obsessive-compulsive about his appearance when he left the house. Kaydee graduated when Mitchell entered eighth grade, and after she left for college, he began to withdraw. He loved going to her college softball games to see her play, and she would come to his games when she could.

I began my research and was away from home a lot during this time, which left David and Mitchell to figure out the details of daily life. They had some good times together, working on the truck and racing go-carts. Looking back, I don't remember Mitchell getting input on anything. He and David seemed to be competing and often butted heads. I put pressure on Mitchell with my selfish expectations as he entered high school. I wanted to attend his football games and events but was absent most of the time, either physically or emotionally. He began to hang out with other kids who were also left to their own devices and decisions. A big red flag went unnoticed. Soon his football buddies stopped coming over, and Mitchell was alone a lot.

Mitchell started smoking marijuana and trying mushrooms between his sophomore and junior year, but it didn't seem to hinder his schoolwork. He showed some decline during his junior year by withdrawing; even so, I still let him fend for himself. Mitchell was brilliant and always kept his grades up, having five math credits before his senior year. He even took his senior English class the summer before his senior year. Then in January of that school year, we faced what should have been a wake-up call.

It's 2015. Mitchell called 9-1-1 to tell them that somebody was coming to kill us. It was my first experience with the local sheriff's department. They came to our home, and when they realized Mitchell's mental state, they had no choice but to take him to the hospital for further evaluation. I was in shock and maybe denial too. I didn't realize what had just happened. I thought perhaps he just took some bad drugs. It seems so weird to me now writing those words as if his drug use was no big deal. I mean really, I question myself. What parent shrugs off their kid's drug use? No mom in her right mind. I did not see this as a red flag and never suspected that it would lead to a complete brain shut down.

Later, when Mitchell came home, things did not improve. He was floating through his school day, not even conscious of where he was, even when he was not doing drugs. I felt this was a temporary teenaged rebellion. I pulled him out of school in

February. Since I had two more countries where I was scheduled to speak, I thought I would take him with me. So, Mitchell got to experience Punta Cana and Norway that Spring. Because of the credits he had earned early, he could still graduate on time with his class.

I began looking for places to send him. I didn't know what to do to help him, so again, I was trying to put him off, put him away, as it were, not taking responsibility. In Colorado, I found Outward Bound a great adventure camp. Mitchell was excited to attend. His communication skills were already slowing down, a key I didn't pick up on at the time. In July of 2015, we sent Mitchell to Colorado. He did not make it a week. They sent him back. Now I realize we have a problem. I did not know how to address it. I was still in the middle of finishing the research I was working on, and I was traveling. Morning Glory Ranch was operating at high speed. We'd just built an equestrian facility, and we were pulling in all kinds of new ABI therapies and treatments. We were moving forward to help every child that walked through our door. The real problem was, I wasn't helping my own.

We floated along and got through January 2016. We put Mitchell in a little camper at the facility to live on his own, which didn't work out. We had to police the people coming onto the property and bringing him drugs. Mitchell was often on drugs and out of control. In May, he had another psychotic break and went to jail. I called the sheriff's office because I thought they would help, but they couldn't assist in the way that Mitchell needed help. There were only two choices. Go to jail or leave my son there in a puddle on the porch. Mitchell went to jail.

I still didn't wake up. It was as if God was saying, "You have to stop what you're doing and focus on your child because he's headed down a big hill in a hurry," My response? "So, okay, he's going to jail." I didn't get it. I was doing those things we declare we'll never do as a parent. I had left him to take care of his own issues, and he didn't know how. Now he is sitting in the county jail. After some finagling, I moved him to a psychiatric hospital to seek more help.

I was selected to travel to Malawi to work with malnourished children in the middle of this. Malawi had the largest population of children dying from malnourishment globally, and I was in a position to make a big difference. So, I left Mitchell in the hands of doctors supporting psychiatry and pharmacology, once again giving him to someone else to deal with his issues.

When I returned from the two weeks in Malawi, I got Mitchell out of the hospital, and our lives continued pretty much the way they had been. Then in October, Mitchell got arrested again for minor drug possession. He was in jail for 15 days. Since he was an adult, I had no recourse to help him. And now, finally, I realize I've got to do something different. Then my girlfriend in California says, "Hey, I've got a program for boys. Why don't you let him come and spend a week or so here?" I quickly said yes, "that would be fantastic, then I could come hang out with you, yada, yada, yada." So, Mitchell and his friend Austin flew to Sacramento in November of 2016 where they could visit my friend's boys' Ranch. And since Mitchell knows ranches, I'm thinking it's going to be a great, comfortable place. There are men counselors, and people who will help him start verbalizing what's going on with him.

Shortly after, I left for Santiago, Chile, to present the last piece of my research to the University of Autonoma. I was done traveling for a while, and I was looking forward to a bit of rest. That's when I got the phone call from my friend in California; Mitchell is catatonic. I got back home and started praying as we do when things hit rock bottom. I asked God right then to help me right now. Fix him. Fix him. Telling God, "Do it now!" All I could think was getting in the car and going to get my son.

At that moment, my world as I knew it stopped. Everything! I quit my research. I let go of every person I was working with, even my family. I realized that this was the time for me to buckle down and do everything I had not done for my child to this point.

It was December 1st, 2016, and Mitchell's brain shut down at nineteen years old.

— Chapter 3 —

FACE-TO-FACE WITH DEEP PRIMAL FEAR

It took 26 hours of driving to get to Sacramento. When I arrived, Mitchell was in the exact shape described by my friend, unable to eat, drink or walk. My heart was devastated seeing my son in this condition. Mitchell's pupils were dilated, which indicated brain injury. I pulled some strings with my professional contacts and got Mitchell in at the UC Davis to get an MRI at a time when it was a seven month wait for the procedure.

Transporting him to the hospital was difficult, but we managed to get him into my car. He was so confused and on high alert with every movement and sound. The next challenge would be getting him into the MRI machine. Let me tell you; it was pure hell. Mitchell screamed and cried; he was punching at everything—he was terrified. He was exhibiting all of the deep primal fear behaviors. He was in survival mode—fight or flight! Everything he saw looked like it was attacking him. All I could do was hold him as tight as I could. He was an emaciated 95 pounds, weak and completely vulnerable, but demonstrating beyond human strength. I kept telling him, "I need you here. We've got you." At that moment, I realized that if he was going to live, it would be up to me. Mitchell was incapable of helping himself.

The MRI came back clear! Nothing was wrong with him—his pressure was good, no lesions, no blood, he's fine. His behavior said otherwise. My brain screamed, "Does he look fine?" I was immediately overcome with guilt, shame, and remorse. I blamed myself for everything, asking all the questions in my head, "How did I do this? Why is this happening? Why God? I've done good work. I've helped children all over the world. Why me? Why

Mitchell? Why does he have to suffer?" It was a hard place where I was bearing the burden of it all.

So, we packed up and started the long drive back to Houston. I was tense and on full alert just like Mitchell; he was like a feral cat, for lack of a better comparison. Any sound could trigger a primal response. I thought that if I could keep him calm until we got to Houston, I'd figure out what I needed to do next. I put on soothing music and tried to travel only during the day. He was hitting himself in the face and head a lot, even slamming his head into the window. He had bruises all over his head and even gave himself a black eye. It was as though his head hurt, and he didn't know how to make it stop. Mitchell never closed his eyes on the entire drive. When we stopped, I'd get food, but he couldn't feed himself as his hand-to-mouth coordination wasn't firing neurologically. I fed him like a toddler. To get him to drink, I had to put the straw in his mouth so that he could suck through the straw. We went through drive-thrus because getting him out of the car was nearly impossible. One fuel stop would take us an hour. I'd take him to the

bathroom, and people were looking at me like, "Do you need help?"
Frankly, I did not know what I needed.

After 17 hours, I needed to sleep but was unsure how that would
work. I rented a bottom-floor corner hotel room so that if we

needed to get out of
there, it would be
easier for Mitchell.
Neither of us rested
well. It was 25 degrees
outside and somehow
the cold seemed to
slow the psychosis
down. We continued
on the next day.

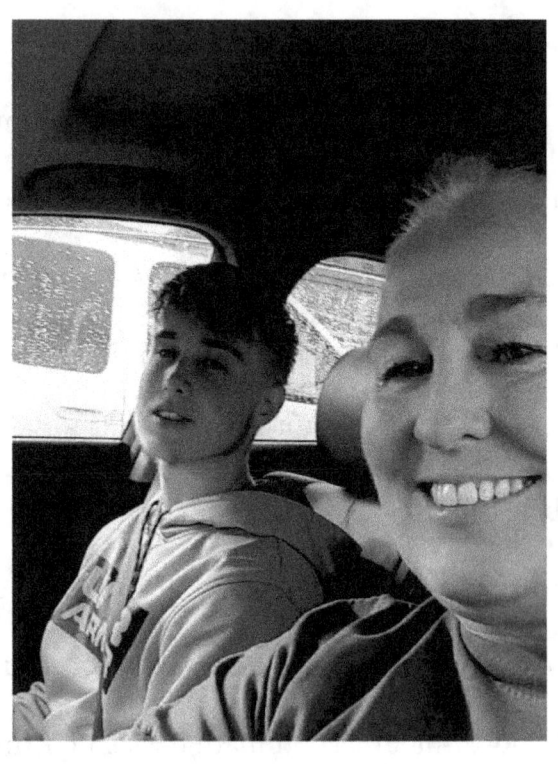

I did a lot of processing while driving. Remember, we were 26
hours and 2000 miles from home. That's a lot of time to think and
run the events through my brain while in a state of high tension.
And I did not know what to expect next from my son. Unpredictable

psychosis is like a war and you are waiting for enemy fire. I'm thinking, "Okay, what have I learned in my research? Where am I? Alright, God, you're going to have to help me here." And I remembered what my great grandmother told me when my first child was about to be born. I'd sit with her and ask, "So, how am I going to know what to do, Granny? I don't know what to do with a baby." And she said, "Honey, you're going to have to surrender and sit there. Pray to Jesus, and He will show you. It'll come to you." I honestly didn't know what she meant until that day with Mitchell in a state of complete helplessness. But that day, her voice rang loud and clear, and it came to me, I need Jesus.

I said the most significant prayer of my life. And I said it out loud where Mitchell could hear it, right there in that car, driving down Interstate 10 in Arizona. It came to me like a flood, and I began to pray. "Jesus, I need you to help me remember what I need to do. I need you to put my momma umbilical cord back on and help me save him." The guilt and shame I had been experiencing seemed to diminish a little. Then I declared, "Alright, Mitchell, we're doing this. Whatever is in there, we're going to get it out. And you're going to be right back here. We're going to do whatever we need to, and you're going to live your best life!" I remember him smiling like he understood me. Still, there was nothing in his eyes that told me he really did understand. His beautiful blue eyes were solid black pupils. His big muscles turned to skin and bone, and his face was tired. He didn't even look like my little boy anymore. But I purposed in my heart then and there, "You are going to live your best life!" And I believed it with my whole being.

It was no easy place we were in at this moment. I took a deep breath and began documenting all the functional responses I had witnessed with Mitchel thus far. I knew I had to track his behaviors to recognize increased functions as they happened no matter how small. God showed me that I had not paid attention to the right things in life. It had been all about my research, finishing each project. It was about other people's children and other families and how I helped them through my research discoveries. I sought to inspire and give hope to them, to the detriment of my child. I had to get real with myself and be raw and deeply honest. It was time for the tables to turn and for me to focus on my family, especially my son. My public research was finished, and my career was on hold. Everything I'd learned shifted and turned inward. I was determined to help my son and to do whatever it took to help him heal and regain the life God had planned for him.

— Chapter 4 —

ROLLING THE DICE

The brutality of our trip back to Texas left us exhausted. All I could think was, "What do we do now?" and "Is there a test that can help us discover the underlying cause of Mitchell's current state? I knew the source of brain activity was electrical firing, so I needed to see the status of Mitchell's neurological connections. Dr. Nancy White, one of the founders of EEG in the 60s who helped develop the technology for measuring brain frequency and electrical output, lived in Houston! I contacted her office on the way back, made an appointment for the test, and drove straight to her office—another blessing of God.

When we arrived at her office, she informed me that Mitchell would be her last patient. She was in her 80s and about to retire! A complete inspiration! She set us up for a highly specific quantitative EEG, revealing extensive information. After an hour of testing, she sat me down with tears in her eyes. Her first question was, "Did he ever play football?" My heart sank. The one-inch-thick stack of colored printouts showed that his occipital and frontal lobes were critical. There were multiple undiagnosed concussions (probably 6 to 10 years old), and the alpha wave frequency he needed for rest and sleep was off the chart. Alone, these concussions would have healed themselves because the brain is quite resilient and placid. However, coupled with his drug use, it caused a full-on functional shut down.

We began him on a schedule of EEGs to document his brain waves. We know that the brain will shut down everything except what is needed for survival, redirecting all its energy to staying alive. The malfunction of his brain activity essentially rewired his brain, bombarding it with different electronic frequencies. Our hope and prayer were that we could reactivate some of the signals in his brain that were not firing adequately. We could see on a monitoring screen what was happening when we tried different frequencies! Thanks to a highly-skilled doctor and technician, we successfully located the areas misfiring and addressed them. After each session, Mitchell seemed calmer and clearer. We did similar treatments at home, which worked for a little while.

I was numb through the entire process. David, who was stressed, tried his best to help us. The constant fear and emotional trauma of not knowing when Mitchell would have a psychotic episode or when you might have to clean your grown child's body and diapers was a huge burden on us both. David took on as much as he could while I searched for answers and treatments. Mitchell would have some semblance of normalcy, then bam, back to psychosis. I could see that David began to resent Mitchell and felt like he was faking his symptoms to manipulate me. David and I disagreed on what to do with Mitchell, and frankly, each other, too.

We were both emotional wrecks. Truth be told, we didn't know what to do.

I'm grabbing at what seemed right, rolling the dice into the unknown. One thing I knew, we had to get Mitchell to shut his eyes. His brain had to rest to heal. I used a product developed in our research that helped regulate Mitchell's alpha waves, allowing him to sleep. Since he had diminished eating ability, we ground his athletic supplements into a powder. Then we put everything into a smoothie so Mitchell could drink it from a straw, which worked. And for the first time, Mitchell laid down and went to sleep. He was home, in his own bed, and he slept for twenty hours!

I researched like a maniac during those twenty hours, going through everything I'd learned. Perhaps Mitchell's condition was drug-induced, so I researched synthetic marijuana and other drugs. At the same time, I was looking at concussion recovery, inflammation, and autoimmune issues. We were trying to regulate Mitchell's brain function. I will go into the science and research of what guided me to my decisions for Mitchell's care in another book.

But for now, I had products that would help his brain, heart, and lung function, it also helped his bones, eyes, and skin. In fact, this one product was doing so many things to keep him healthy systemically that I quadrupled the dosage!

I also learned how to detox his body from heavy metals from drug use that could cause inflammation and stop concussions from repairing. We had a lot of work to do, but this was the most logical scientific roll of the dice I had ever done. Our biggest concern was that his body would stay healthy long enough to allow complete healing.

We had done well with Mitchell's nutrition. Now I focused on gut health. The gut is a direct line to the brain. I learned from my studies that the gut manages attacks from anything outside our environment. We have what's called gut flora, gut bacteria, gut viruses, and gut life that keep our bodies healthy. The health condition of our gut is constantly changing, modifying, and adjusting. I knew of a product that was having great success. Through my professional connections, I got a six-month supply from our China Innovation Center and put pro and prebiotics into Mitchell's nutrition protocol. I monitored even the slightest change we observed in him, making careful notes of functional improvement.

Next, I began to bring in specialists to the Ranch who might offer us help: occupational and physical therapists, chiropractors,

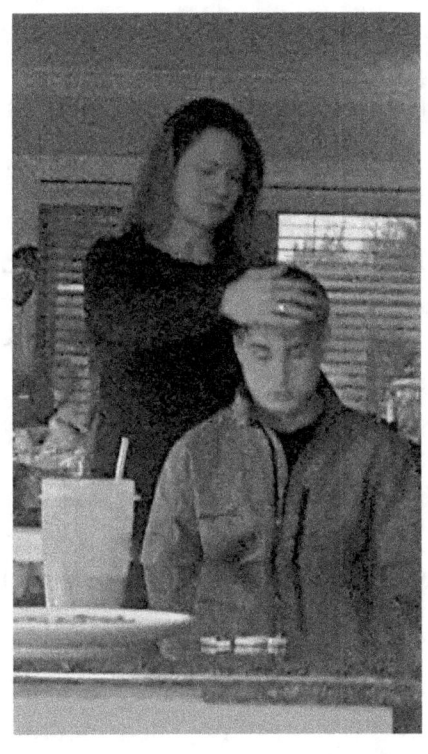

a cranial specialist, Dr. Cari DeSchmidt, as well as an incredible ophthalmologist Dr. Marcia Smith. We added massage therapy four times a week. It was a grueling schedule, but by the end of February 2017, Mitchell could put food in his mouth. We were moving forward. It was exciting and validating. All of my struggles were worth it. The therapies that produced progress gave me hope. I had a prayer and a dream that this would be the magic wand that would connect Mitchell's brain so that I would have my baby back.

Every step had been indescribably difficult. Mitchell's unforeseeable behaviors continued throughout 2017 and into early 2018. We were all under intense stress, not wanting to make a wrong move to set Mitchell off. He would break windows, punch walls (or us!), pull doors off hinges, pick up and throw anything he could get his hands on in a rage. David often felt like Mitchell was trying to kill him.

I failed to realize how much pressure I placed on my husband. David drove Mitchell to and from his neurofeedback treatments, which was a huge blessing. Toward the end of February, traveling 70 mph down Interstate 10 on their way home, Mitchell tried to jump out of the truck. My husband did everything he could to keep him from falling onto the highway, managing to pull him back inside. Then Mitchell tried it again. In a state of a near nervous breakdown, David pulled over on a country road, put Mitchell out of the truck, and left him there. Of course, I panicked. I couldn't find Mitchell. I didn't know what to do. Someone from a local shop called me saying Mitchell wandered in. He rattled off my phone number when they asked if they could help him. I thank God that he remembered it and relayed it to those who could help him. That day, Mitchell's behavior was the straw that broke the camel's back as far as David was concerned. From then on, David took a supporting role away from us—to survive and preserve his sanity. We rented Mitchell a house in town so that David wouldn't leave, but that didn't work out. David took a permanent break from our situation in late March and moved out. Later, I realized that I didn't give him enough credit for all he did for us in the years I traveled extensively. On top of that, three extreme months after Mitchell's shutdown. It was more than he could take.

I couldn't see it at the time, and I was furious about his actions and resentful of everybody. I was hurt, anxious, and afraid. David had been the only person holding me together. Now I had no idea how I would handle Mitchell's care on my own. My husband, my rock, was gone. I focused on my role as mama. I was alone, but I was determined to get Mitchell stronger.

I learned how to handle stress alone and found a way to treat Mitchell's condition like another piece of research. As we moved through the first year of hard, intensive survival, I put Mitchell in a protective bubble. We created a dark environment with no lights, sound, visitors, or noise in our house. We were isolated. Through it, my brain went in every direction to resolve where I was with my son.

I learned something that would become the most powerful part of my research; there's only so far you can go with man's research. After that point, it's only God! I call that the God Gap—the unknown space where you pray, have faith, love, and live in a positive environment. It's the space where love comes in and healing begins. I learned the hard way; I could only do so much. God had to handle the rest of it.

Even with the improvements Mitchell made, I observed more unpredictable psychoses daily. He was hallucinating. I finally thought to play into the psychosis with him. It was a scary place, and being a little bit of a daredevil in my youth, I felt like I could learn more about his hallucinations if I jumped in to play along. It was a danger zone that turned into a love zone. He was getting stronger, and although the frequency of the events diminished, the intensity grew to be more significant. I likened these episodes to experiencing a live video game of intense interaction. Every daytime nightmare blackout had been the same. He became very verbal saying, the phrases repeatedly during every episode, but this one was different. He kept saying, "They killed Opi; they are killing Margo and Christine!" I interacted with him, asking him questions like, "What weapon are they using? Where is Opi? Let's save them. I've got your back!" When he realized he had backup, he stopped. He looked at me with the most painful expression. Then he hugged me tight as I whispered in his ear that Opi (his grandfather), Margo, (his aunt), and Christina (his cousin) were okay. He spoke with them by phone to reassure him that they and he were alright. He was stuck in a daytime nightmare about someone hurting the people he loved. I couldn't help but think to myself, "Maybe there is a hell gap, too."

It was heart-wrenching watching him wake up from that nightmare. He had so much fear that he could hardly move. He would repeat to me, "I didn't do that. I didn't do it." I reassured him it was okay, and then we cleaned up. But each time, his shame over the things he would destroy kept compounding. He didn't know why or how it happened. I wanted to help him overcome those emotions. I learned that the only way to tackle shame is with empathy. So, I searched for people who possessed this character trait. We also still had the equine therapy facility and our horses, the most magical, unconditional loving animals on the planet, and they possess empathy. I surrounded Mitchell with empathetic people, he was interacting with the horses, but the damage had been done. He was no longer speaking.

I addressed physical and nutritional needs, but I learned it was all in the God Gap when it came to the emotional realm of wellness. There was nothing more I could do. I realized there's only brain health and the God Gap. And the only way I can change any of

Mitchell's brain functions is to improve his brain's health, give him unconditional love, and pray without ceasing. We were back to where we had started months ago. Soon we would increase movement and add lifestyle medicine too. We weren't quite there by the fourth quarter of 2017. We couldn't foresee that another disaster lay just ahead of us.

— Chapter 5 —

EARTHLY ANGELS ALIGHT

Earlier in 2017, I hired a young man, Meshak, to be a companion caregiver for Mitchell. He was a unique spiritual and biblical man who played football at Texas A&M, Prairie View. He was strong enough to protect himself from Mitchell's rages and possessed the empathy Mitchell needed. He was also a great blessing to me, transporting Mitchell to appointments and events. He and Mitchell lived in a small house in town for a bit, but I quickly realized that would not work. Mitchell needed wide-open spaces to roam, run, and swim in the ponds. He also needed a safe area during blackout episodes.

Morning Glory Ranch was still operating, and my staff, praise God, was holding it together the best they could without me being there, without David, and without any input or financial support.

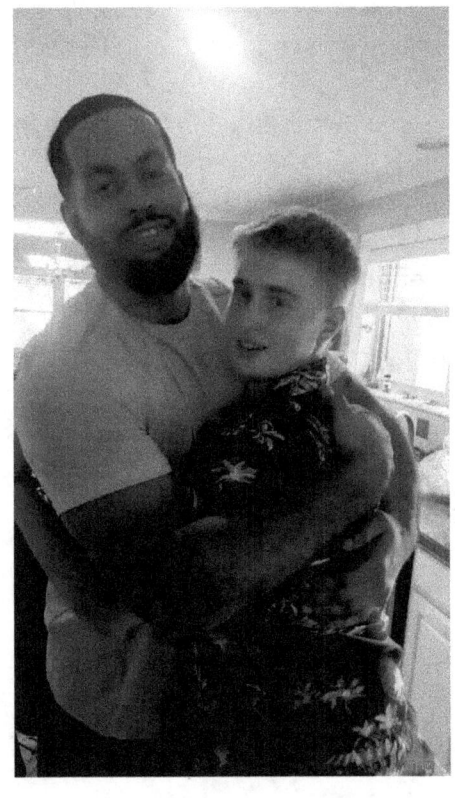

The Ranch was my baby, my dream. I founded the organization and built the 45,000 square foot facility through donors who had partnered with my research and nutritional products that were supporting brain health around the world. I was passionate about offering the same therapies we were discovering for Mitchell under one roof so that our clients could avoid the trauma of going place-to-place for treatments that ultimately would be in-effective. So, as we made our plans for implementation, we also decided to build

Mitchell an 1800 square foot house inside the arena. While we built the home, I had to ensure that Mitchell was never by himself. In hindsight, that seemed to be when fear set in, resulting in the chaos, destruction, and mayhem I described before. Meshak was a godsend during this time. His presence gave me the relief I needed to sleep, knowing Mitchell was in his own home with support for a few hours. I tried to decompress, but I was stressed to the max, working to pay the bills, juggling family, and dealing with the real possibility of having to shut the charity down. Mitchell and Meshak moved in as soon as the house was complete.

Mitchell was making progress once again. When he was lucid, he tried to be productive. He tried to help with the horses and even started cooking. There were sparks of the old Mitchell coming through, and my heart was so happy to see him thrive. Even if it was small, it was a win to me.

On December 16, 2017, at 10:15 a.m., Meshak left for class, and there was supposed to be another therapist there by 10. I was at my house across the pasture cooking for the day. I still had a few staff coming in to help with the horses, and I got a call from one of them saying Mitchell's apartment was on fire. I raced down there to find my son trapped in the fire. My staff had already called the fire department, and I could hear the sirens blaring as they drew close to the Ranch.

Adrenaline hit me hard and fast. I was like a mom whose baby is trapped under the car who, through superhero strength, picks up a two-ton vehicle. I kicked the front door open only to see too much flame to get to him. I went around to kick the back door open, still too much fire and smoke. Mitchell is screaming, "Mom! Mom! Help me! You have to get me, Mom!" Even to this day, I can hear his cries. I ran around to the bedroom window, the only access left. It was only a 24 by 24-inch window built into the metal building. I see Mitchell. He's covered in black soot, raging flames behind him. I busted out that window and told him to jump! I yelled, "You have to jump! You have to jump NOW, Son!" Yet all I could hear him say was, "Mommy, mommy, help me, help me! You have to get me."

With smoke roiling up his back, Mitchell is solid black, and flames are on the bed right behind him. I pleaded, "Please, God, don't let my son die in this fire!" Mitchell finally came to the window. I grabbed him and pulled him through. When Mitchell stood up, he was like a wild, caged animal. He started swinging and running and hitting everything he could within his reach. At this point, some of the firemen and EMTs had arrived, and they were helping me get him under control. The ambulance was there, and all I could think was that I had to know how much smoke he had inhaled. It was one of the most terrifying events of our lives. And, to this day, I am terrified of fire! I believe that Mitchell was in pure hell that day, and this fire, engulfing an 1800 square foot home, trapping my son, was the devil's last attempt to take him out.

At this point, on this day, after a year of struggle and heartache and doing everything in my own strength, devaluing my family by putting them on the backburner, doing all I could discover for Mitchell, I finally surrendered everything and everyone to God. I completely let go. Our lives were in His hands, and I felt an unexpected release from all my fear, anxiety, chaos, struggle, bitterness, and exhaustion. I felt an unfamiliar sensation of a peace that I knew was God's peace. I finally entered—spirit, soul, and body—the God Gap on December 16, 2017.

Mitchell needed to go to the hospital, but getting him on the gurney was not an easy task. The EMTs and I got him calmed down enough to get him strapped down. I can tell you, seeing your kid strapped down on a gurney, covered in black soot, is an image you can never unsee.

The medical staff pumped him full of anti-anxiety drugs at the hospital, x-rayed and evaluated him, and reported back that he was fine, with no smoke inhalation. Praise God! However, they had to keep him strapped down. I snapped a few pictures of him in my nervous energy at the hospital. The way he was looking at me was oddly angelic. He has this mommy saved me look, filled with a unique look of love I've ever seen. It was almost like he died and came back. He was looking at me like a little boy in awe of his mother.

The hospital social services staff tried to find a "good"

psychiatric ward (if there even is such a thing) for Mitchell. A police officer guarded the door as my little caged animal was ready to run. He'd taken a couple of laps around the hospital floor when no one was watching him. The hospital would only keep him for 72 hours. Unable to find an appropriate mental health facility for Mitchell, we brought him home.

Mitchell and Meshak had no place to live, so they moved into the house across the pasture, my home. Meshak left us at the end of his semester and went home, so now it was just Mitchell and Mom—again.

After much lamenting, I decided to suspend operations at Morning Glory Ranch to reevaluate where we were. My staff was some of the most creative and loving human beings I knew. They gave their hearts and souls to our kids and their families, and I'll always be grateful. Ending it broke my heart, yet at the same time, brought relief. My life was pivoting again; however, I was pivoting this time in the God Gap completely surrendered.

Christmas was almost here, and I had presents to wrap. Some

girls came over to help. They gave Mitchell lots of love and attention. He enjoyed himself, and it made my heart so happy to see him smile and light up the room. He was still on anti-anxiety medication from the hospital. It was the first time he had been on pharmaceutical drugs. The medical staff pumped him full of drugs

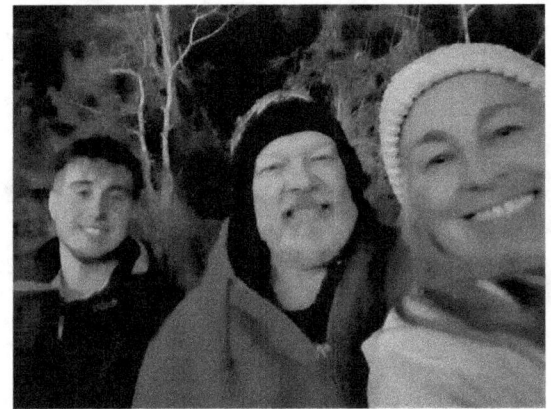

during his hospital stay, and they seemed to be working, even temporarily. Mitchell was doing well.

The day after our wonderful time wrapping gifts and receiving visitors, David and I thought we would take Mitchell to the Festival of Lights in College Station, Santa's Wonderland. The lights and decorations were so beautiful; we had a great time. We had our boy back! He smiled and laughed, ate dinner with us, and sat on rides and hayrides. It was magical, like seeing your six-or-seven-year-old child in awe of Christmas wonder. What a gift—a gift from God.

We were at peace for the first time in years. I felt God covering us, holding us together, and leading the way. As the sun began to set, it did not occur to me that the lights would create different types of images for Mitchell in the darkness. I forgot about that part of his condition in the beauty of our day.

Mitchell drifted away from us, it got dark, and his fear (fight or flight) center kicked in. The next thing I knew, he was arrested for punching a lady at the park. NOT AGAIN! He was taken to the Brazos County Jail. I'm panicking. I didn't know what to do, just trying to breathe, which was difficult.

The only saving grace was that through our work at Morning Glory Ranch, lawyers, district attorneys, and law enforcement officers in College Station knew of our work. Now I had to have faith in God, believing that, this time, someone would help us.

First, the County Judge, Amanda Matzke, was incredible. Judge Matzke assigned *angel* attorney, Mark Maltsberger, who took Mitchell's case pro bono. He specialized in unique Texas cases like Mitchell's, so his legal help would make a difference in Mitchell's life. Mark spent hours working directly with the court and the District Attorney's office to see that Mitchell had no charges filed. He also stayed by our side until Mitchell was home in June. Mark continues to support us through love and prayer. And I believe we have inspired him to become a judge to help more families like ours. And it did. He and Judge Matzke were the first people I believe God set in motion for us.

Our interaction in her Court was the first event I believe God set in motion for us. I considered her an *angel* too. As ugly, nasty, and painful as this situation was, Judge Matzke was God's saving grace. I remember her saying, "Kim, I will keep Mitchell by himself with two deputies, so he's protected. And they'll play basketball with him 24/7 until I can get you guardianship. You have to be able to protect him." Her ability to see what Mitchell needed most was a miracle. In every other incident, Mitchell's condition was disregarded, so he was handled strictly as an adult, which never got him the desperately needed help and protection required. I felt a sense of peace and hope finally. I was still scared for Mitchell, but

I had let God take over. I counted this moment as surrender number three on our journey.

The next *angel* on the scene was Kit Wright, who was in charge of the jail's medical system, who is now a very close friend. She took a very special interest in Mitchell, saying, "I see kids in my jail with these types of functions all the time, but you're the only mom that's doing anything about it. What are you doing?" Kit gave Mitchell his supplements and called me every day. She messaged me to tell me how my boy was doing until Judge Matzke could fast-track guardianship for me so that when he came out of that jail, I would have legal recourse to protect him. I felt like everything was changing for the better at this point. I heard of so many moms whose ABI children ended up in jail, became homeless, or who were nowhere to be found, or worse, committed suicide. All because parents could not get guardianship. It was a major turning point in our lives. Now I could get Mitchell out of jail without charges and into a neuro-rehabilitation facility. It had taken over two months, but on March 1, 2018, he was transferred to a medical facility. And the first thing they did was pump him full of psychiatric meds. Mitchell was on pharmaceutical drugs again. Something that would later prove to be the worst mistake for his ultimate healing. It's only a temporary band aid, not a long-term solution for independent living.

— Chapter 6 —

THE MARTIAL NANNIES

Finally, we knew we found a suitable facility while Mitchell was still in jail in Brazos County; however, the costs were exorbitant. While I made good money, $2,000 a day was out of the question! Mark Maltsberger, Mitchell's court-appointed attorney and a good friend, began researching to find a more cost-effective treatment facility.

I started researching the insurance offered that might fit Mitchell's condition. Only catastrophic policies covered brain injuries written explicitly as an acquired brain injury or diagnosed autism at birth. Thankfully, with that first quantitative EEG conducted by Dr. Nancy White, his condition was listed as an acquired brain injury. We gathered all the test results to get a temporary catastrophic policy covering brain injury. When we finally got Mitchell transferred, the insurance company refused to cover his care two weeks later, forcing me to retain an insurance attorney. Mitchell was admitted to Nexus Neurorecovery Center, one of America's best neuro rehab facilities, where we were grateful to meet another *angel*, Dr. Cassady.

Soon after, the insurance company tried to deny coverage, stating that behaviors were a mental health issue. I had learned that behaviors are the result of brain health. I set out to find the research that would support my thesis that there is no such thing as "mental health," only brain health that directly results from a malfunction of the cells in your brain. It felt like a losing battle.

While I had to force the issue, thankfully, the Nexus staff gave Mitchell the nutritional supplements that worked well for him in the past. They continued to administer pharmaceuticals, lots of them, which required weekly bloodwork to monitor levels of toxins in his system. Mitchell's good nutrition kept those levels manageable. Ninety days later, he left the facility with 10,000 to 15,000 milligrams of drugs, per day, being pumped into his body. Now he was sick. Pharmaceutical sick.

I knew I needed a plan for him when he came home, and those 90 days gave me time to set it up. God and the Texas court system gave me guardianship of my son, and at last, I felt we had a chance to help him stay safe and recover.

My research led to developing a movement protocol that would address Mitchell's behaviors, which gave me peace and hope! I knew the Holy Spirit was on the move in our lives. I wholeheartedly believed we would win and that Mitchell would have his life back.

Everyone I looked to for help almost immediately showed up, even folks I could have never imagined. Finally, a light at the end of the tunnel! I had no idea what our exact path might look like or how long it was going to take. After five months of being away, Mitchell came home.

The way God orchestrated what happened over the next few months was incredible; some events and connections demonstrated to me once again, every second of my existence is Divinely planned.

Let me share a bit about them with you. I met John Koko on a company trip in January of 2012. He was a highly renowned acupuncturist and taught his craft at schools nationwide. He also had a son on the autism spectrum and had taken great interest in Morning Glory Ranch. John wanted to film a documentary at MGR, and while producing it brought a lot of people into my life. I met Jesse through John. Jesse introduced me to Marilyn Cooper. They were trained in Kung Fu, Tai Chi, and Medical Qigong. Marilyn was quite interested in what we were doing at the Ranch. On a visit, she told us about her protégé Javier Rodriguez from San Antonio, who worked with Yang's Martial Arts Association (YMAA) and its founder, Dr. Yang, Jwing-Ming. Javier was an expert in martial arts. Soon he and his girlfriend Nona visited the Ranch. They loved it.

As Mitchell's exit from rehab approached, I decided to call

Javier to see if he would consider living with us for a few months. I wanted him to help wean Mitchell off his medications and teach him, Tai Chi. Javier was quickly all in with our plan, which was fantastic. He was a 100% God-sent *angel*.

Mitchell was so excited. He was functioning very well on all that pharma, except for the side effects of bloating, constipation, sleeplessness, and drooling! He was able to speak words and move more fluidly. The erratic psychoses 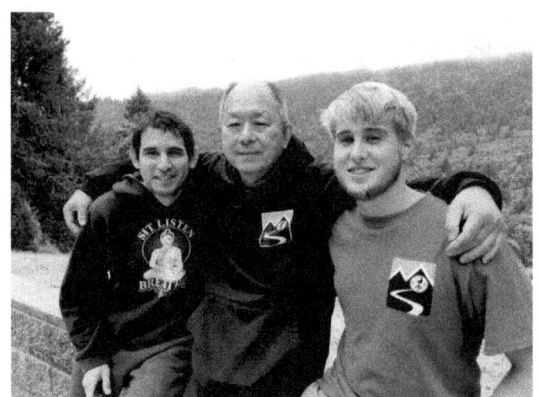 were shorter in duration but now more intense.

Mitchell's physical functioning was better; however, it was much more dangerous and destructive when he went into an unpredictable blackout. We could be driving down the road having a great time, then suddenly Mitchell is punching the windshield out!

I couldn't do it anymore. I had a hunch that the

pharmaceuticals were the culprit, so I decided to wean him off the medication. During the process, I increased his nutritional supplementation.

While Mitchell was still highly functional, I took him and Javier on a business trip to Bermuda. Mitchell had a great time: Tai Chi on the pink sand beaches, jet-skiing around the island, snorkeling sunken ships, and receiving lots of love from my team from around the world. It was a wonderful experience and opportunity for regrowing brain cells and building self-worth. He only had a couple of blackout moments, but the people around helped Mitchell pull through each one.

Javier couldn't stay forever, so after witnessing the effects of surrounding Mitchell with loving support, he decided that we needed a group of compassionate experts to help in Mitchell's recovery. I'll never forget the moment Javier said, "Let's get a team in here!" Javi, as I playfully called him, contacted everyone we knew at YMMA, whom we thought would be a great fit for team Mitchell. His decision was indeed a blessing; it was again a God Gap moment. Javier called up some of the best martial arts people he knew. We needed what I termed martial arts nannies who could

defend and take care of themselves while keeping Mitchell safe and from being destructive. It was perfect! I also thought it would benefit future ABI clients, so we started a new business, WHOListic Brain Health Village, Inc. It was then I knew we only heal in community.

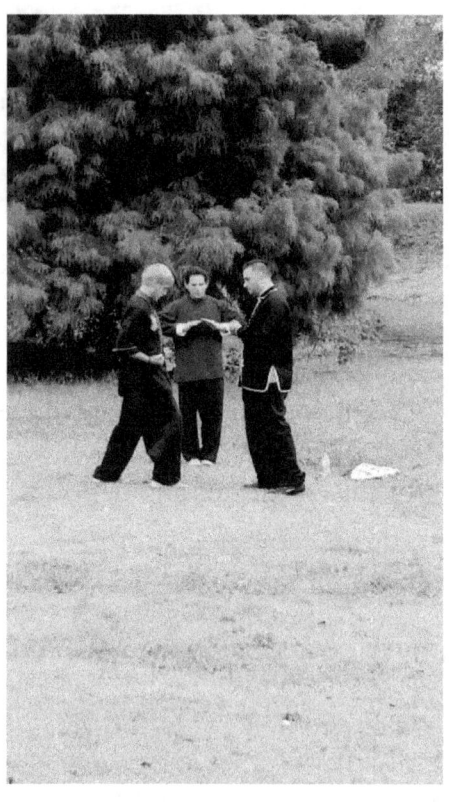

Javier brought in six or seven guys to see how they would work out as they interacted with Mitchell. They stayed at the house while they were there. We were all living in the farmhouse because the home inside the facility was under renovation due to the fire. One of the *martial nannies*, Jonathan, was a Sifu, an incredible Kung Fu artist, a big guy from Yonkers, NY. Jonathan came down every weekend to work with Mitchell for eight months, sometimes staying for an entire week. Mitchell advanced as he learned Kung Fu (up to 7 levels).

Now it's late fall, and we had a team of four young men working diligently with Mitchell. Jacob came on board in October and proved himself to be an absolute God-sent *angel*. He supported me in marvelous ways, even giving me a shoulder to cry on from time to time. He was invaluable to both my son and me, offering support beyond what was required. He wrapped Mitchell up in so much love as we approached the wellness he needed to achieve. His words ring in my heart, "We're not putting Mitchell back on that crap (the meds). We will rebuild him slow and steadily. No matter how long it takes." He meant it, and to a mom who was starving for answers, Jacob's words were like a healing balm.

Oddly, something significant always seemed to happen in December. This year Mitchell had the most outrageous nightmare ever. However, there was something different about this one. He appeared to be conscious through most of it, and we did not try to stop him. It was interesting when he finally quit. We noted that he chose what he was going to break, and he didn't break anything that meant something to me—pictures, my piano, my things. In the past, he was like a tornado with no ability to decide what he would destroy. It was so interesting to me. I can't explain it entirely, but I had a sense of knowing that this would be the last episode he would ever have. I recognized the Holy Spirit's voice saying, "*This is it!*"

— Chapter 7 —

CONNECTING
THE DOTS

Mitchell's final December blackout caused significant regression in his behaviors, and by January of 2019, it was as though he were three years old again. The loss of function was severe. We had to put food in his mouth, his language was gone, and his toilet skills were non-existent. It was disheartening to see him lose all the ground we had so painstakingly gained.

Jacob and I decided to bring on two additional martial nannies. They were short-lived but helped us manage as we rethought Mitchell's overall wellness and recovery plan. Javier was still putting together protocols and practices; however, he eventually had to go back to YMAA to teach. That left Jacob and me pulling Mitchell up by the bootstraps. We learned that we could do it!

Our most significant discovery was learning that when a person with an acquired brain injury has an enraged blackout, the degeneration in the brain is identical to what results in Parkinson's disease. I was now on another research trail, and God revealed what I needed to focus on in this season. It had to do with dopamine levels, and I used what I learned to adjust Mitchell's nutritional regimen again. I continued researching the effects of dopamine on the brain and how it relates to psychoses. While we know a lot, I learned that there is much that we do not understand that can only be revealed in the God Gap. Through it all I felt the grace of the Holy Spirit leading me over mountains of research, giving me insights that impact not only my son, but many who are challenged by "monsters" termed schizophrenia, ADHD, bi-polar disorder, autism, Parkinson's, Alzheimer's, PTSD and the like. It was groundbreaking research that I'll write about in my next book.

As I connected the dots, Jacob and I went to work applying what we had learned. We modified Mitchell's nutritional protocols and monitored his behaviors as he began to make progress. We made an educated guess, rolled the logical set of dice, and trusted how the Holy Spirit was leading us in the God Gap.

The second phase was bringing back the movement medicine, so Tai Chi breathwork is where Jacob started. It was beautiful seeing the result as we got more oxygen into Mitchell's body by expanding his breathing. We have learned that people with acquired brain injuries do not breathe efficiently. They take shallow breaths, not working the diaphragm, thereby not getting enough oxygen to the brain because oxygen does not get into the lower lobes of the lungs. It was beautiful to watch Jacob, Jonathan, Javier, and a few other guys lead Mitchell in breathwork. As his breathing improved, we observed him becoming more cognizant every day. God created our brain to give us signals to breathe. When those signals didn't work, it was like I could sense God breathing air into my Mitchell, giving him that source of life.

Everything we do with our body requires brain function. Our brain is like a switchboard. We learned a lot about the benefits of movement in our equine therapy program; we knew its vast effect on the whole body. We got Mitchell to move from the Tai Chi, which required his brain to first fire or connect to tell the body to move. First, basic physical movement like raising his arms, then running, and even swimming in the ponds on the property. Jacob, Javier, and Jonathan worked with Mitchell. Before Jonathan returned to

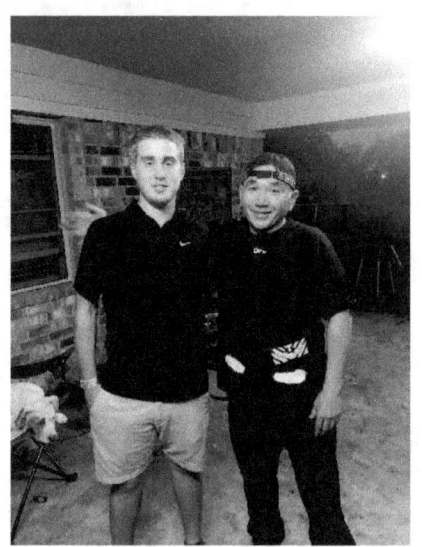

New York, he found Master Quan, a local Kung Fu instructor. He quickly became one of Mitchell's "saviors" and brought prayer back into Mitchell's life, all the while helping him remember his Kung Fu moves.

We enjoined nutritional and movement protocols; Mitchell was getting better. He was functioning at the level of an eight to ten-year-old, but his speech was still lacking. Soon we met yet another

angel, this one from the mountains of Utah.

Adam was an emotional and body language specialist by

vocation. He was skilled at assisting people with using their words,

communicating their feelings, and saying the words they mean so

that the brain could deal with any experienced trauma. So, he was

keenly aware of what Mitchell was feeling. We know that when we

pray, God answers, and God indeed sent Adam with the much-

needed emotional language component. He got to know Mitchell

over several months then asked if Mitchell could go to Utah with

him to camp, kayak, and hike in the mountains. I thought it was

fantastic, especially since Mitchell could toilet himself and do

bodily care like showers with prompting.

Most importantly, the unpredictable psychoses were gone. This

invitation came at a perfect time. David and I were selling the

Ranch in Waller, TX, living in an RV, and praying about our next

step. Mitchell and I flew to Utah in July of 2019 and stayed with

Adam for a few days. It was great to get Mitchell into new

adventures and surroundings, which we knew would help his brain improve. Mitchell loved the mountains and was best at hiking and kayaking. Adam related that he had several emotional releases and believed the variation of oxygen levels between high and low altitudes profoundly affected Mitchell. Adam's determination to help Mitchell brought great benefits. It was a remarkable experience.

Mitchell remained in Utah with Adam until June of 2020, but family events in the early part of that year proved to profoundly impact all of us, especially Mitchell.

— Chapter 8 —

I LOVE YOU, GRANDMA

It's 2020 now, and my mother is very sick. She lived with us for four years at the end of her life, witnessing Mitchell go through many heartaches and struggles. Mom knew how hard life was for me. And she knew how much Mitchell was suffering. As she drew close to death in March, her family and close friends came to say their goodbyes. While everyone else knew she was about to graduate to heaven, Mitchell had no idea. He had been in Utah since July of 2019. My heart was hurting at the thought of losing my mom and from the realization that Mitchell couldn't say goodbye. His grandmother was one of the few people who were always there for him. I had no idea how he was feeling, but I knew he felt the emotional gravity of it all.

My mother was in comfort care, receiving morphine every couple of hours. She'd been here for longer than anyone thought, hanging on for something or someone. I remember the nurses asking if mom had any unfinished business. We were all numb and exhausted; our brains were foggy. The only thing we could think of was that she and

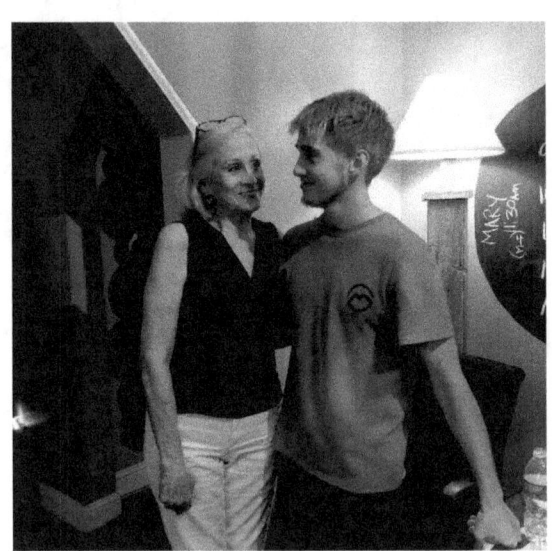

Mitchell had not been able to say goodbye to each other. I didn't realize it then, but the nurses were asking, because they too thought she'd be gone by this time.

It wasn't long after this conversation that mom woke up out of a should have already left this world state and said, "I haven't talked to Mitchell yet." I fell to my knees and cried, "Praise God." I called immediately to track him down. I didn't know what mountain he might be camping on or where he might be hiking. But in a matter of minutes, God found him for us. I got him on the phone, realizing that he didn't talk but knowing that he understands everything he hears. My sister recorded the conversation to have it for Mitchell later if he wanted to listen to it again. I gave the phone to my mother.

"Mitchell," she began, "you get yourself well and take care of your mother. I'm going to heaven now. And I love you." Then to all our surprise, Mitchell responded, "I love you, Grandma." I broke down and cried the hardest I've ever cried. I was on my knees, thanking God for allowing that beautiful moment to happen. Very shortly afterward, my mom went to heaven. Saying goodbye to Mitchell was indeed her unfinished business. Since that day in March, I believe my mother's influence still impacts him, and greater than that, God is watching over him, and day-by-day bringing his healing to completion.

By April 2020, Adam and I searched for testing to see why Mitchell was still not regaining his speech. All our other approaches are solid and consistent—nutritional and movement medicine streamlined. The unpredictable episodes are gone. It is time to design a lifestyle medicine protocol and see if this would help awaken Mitchell's speech.

While Mitchell was in Utah, David and I began looking for where we might move. The MGR facility had been sold, and we bought a little cabin in Willis, TX, near the grandkids and moved in April. During that time, Jacob had sugested looking for a more permanent place around Nacogdoches, TX. We needed to buy another farm where Mitchell could live out in the open, and honestly, I also preferred that. My sister and her family lived in that area; we had strengthened our relationship since our mother passed away. I loved the area and the people.

By summer, Adam's situation in Utah changed due to Covid lockdowns, which dictated Mitchell's return home. They surprised me on my birthday, June 3, making it one of my best birthdays ever, especially since I had only seen Mitchell twice since he went to Utah. The separation had been good for us both, breaking some of the codependency we had developed. The time apart also got us out of our little bubble and encouraged me to believe we were going to make it. I had given everything to God and done what He guided me to do. Our times were in His Hands.

David and I were still looking for real estate in Nacogdoches. It had been a year and a half since I set an alert on my phone for any ranch properties newly listed on the MLS. We looked at a few places, but an alert popped up on the day Mitchell came home. It was a ranch with 27 acres and three houses. One of the things Mitchell verbalized to Adam in Utah was he wanted to live on his own. Adam helped Mitchell plan what he needed to do to make that happen. We knew Mitchell needed a place of his own to begin his lifestyle medicine. I put a contract on the property sight-unseen that same day. We bought a farm that had been in the family for generations. The property had been on the market for only two hours! And, get this, the parents who owned the farm helped underprivileged children and families, and they were loving and kind to Mitchell. We remain friends to this day.

In August, we moved into our ranch home. It was beautiful, overlooking serene ponds, grazing cattle, and always seemed to be cooled by a steady breeze. I knew that this was indeed the place God planned for our future. We named our ranch Heaven's Hill— our happy, healing ranch. Here we would surrender, sit still, and let God work.

Now Mitchell could live alone in one of the homes on the Ranch. Setting things up with him felt good like we were decorating a college dorm. He was learning to be his own person. His progress seemed steady as he recovered his sense of identity. When he had moments of fear, I let him sleep on our couch, but we kept healthy boundaries, especially since David and I were restoring our marriage. We believed God was moving through Mitchell every minute and guiding me to where I needed to be in this season of my life. I was waiting on God to reveal to me what to do next. Mitchell was living on his own, relearning how to take care of his laundry, clean his house and make his food. We allowed God to move us forward in His timing and I am rejoicing as I regain my son.

Soon after moving to Heaven's Hill, we began building community in our new town. My sister introduced me to a much-needed Bible study course. We were living a life of gratitude like never before. We were reacquainting ourselves with Jesus, and the Holy Spirit led me to recommit my life to the Lord. I was baptized again, this time with true conviction in my heart. We became involved in a local church, where our new friends reached out to Mitchell in loving ways. I was overwhelmed by them at times. Empathy surrounded us as God blessed us every day.

Mitchell's function seemed to plateau by September. We thought perhaps the move, and increased expectations of living on his own were impacting his progress. I changed his nutritional protocol once again and continued to monitor him closely. At this point, I started to grow weary and felt I was running out of combinations. We finished the new barn to move the therapy horses to the Ranch by October. Mitchell had grown up with these horses and loved them throughout his life. He had also helped hundreds of other ABI children ride, and I knew that if Mitchell were involved with them again, it would be therapeutic for him to help him remember and rebuild neuropathways.

I bought a new custom horse trailer with living quarters to haul our big Harley Clydesdale and double as a camper for the boys in November. Mitchell and Jacob went camping and kayaking here in East Texas, where many great lakes exist. Mitchell learned to kayak in Utah and was good. On his first outing here, he went all the way across the lake by himself. The winds were too strong for Mitchell to make it back by himself, so Jacob found some boaters who could give him a ride back across, which was a great experience for building problem-solving skills and strength. Our movement medicine program was in full force now, and the boys were working out more to increase strength.

A friend established a community for adults who suffered from psychotic episodes that provided small cabins where they could live independently with a community commissary for eating, a library, and a church, all on-site. Jacob and Mitchell visited often and volunteered. Once more residents moved to the community, it occurred to me that I desired Mitchell to be around people that he could emulate. He needed to be with people recovering from their injuries, seeing progress and growth. Our brain grows and connects based on what it is exposed to, so I began to be very specific in my daily prayers, asking God for a different direction.

Christmases were always hard with Mitchell. He had no concept of day or time, still growing in his communication skills. It had been five years of Christmases, but this year seemed harder since it was our first Christmas without my mother. She was our rock— Mitchell's favorite person. I felt like an orphan, left to do and process all of this independently. I depended on Jesus more now than ever. I found peace with my journey here on earth—me and Jesus. Every day I grew stronger, once again recognizing I had to fight for Mitchell. This time it felt different, more peaceful, like I was in sync with the current of life. There were times I believe the heavenly angels picked me up and carried me around. It was so real.

Even with all of Mitchell's progress, I could feel that something wasn't yet right. We ran lots of tests. Each came back normal and healthy. Mitchell was losing weight, his focus was diminishing, and his speed slowed, which was not expected. It seemed we were on a path we had traveled before. By the end of the year, Mitchell's function and labs were even lower than they had been in June. He was in a critical state. His nutrition absorption levels were plateauing. In October, they began to plummet. By December, he was at the lowest antioxidant absorption that he had ever been. We had a serious problem. Without cell protection, his body was exposed to all kinds of sickness or disease.

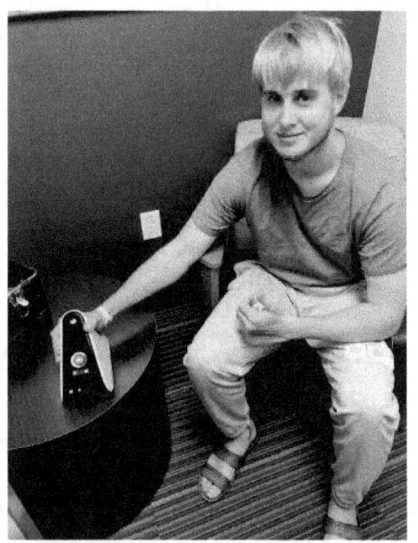

We needed help. *Again.*

— Chapter 9 —

WE CAN FIX IT

The first snow-mageddon hit Texas in January of 2021, and it was a big deal. Our little farmhouse was built by hand, and while it didn't look like much, we appreciated that it had been lovingly constructed by skilled craftsmen at that time and was at least efficient. However, it wasn't built for snowstorms. There is something very magical and peaceful about a heavy snowfall. And since he had lived in the snowy mountains of Utah, Mitchell loved it, and we all just wrapped up in its beauty and enjoyed our time. The peace that we experienced at Heaven's Hill was even more tangible when it was covered in the serene silence of snow.

Then in February, snow-mageddon hit again, and it was much more intense than the first. Our old farmhouse had a propane leak somewhere in the ancient gas lines, and soon, with the power out, we had no heat. The temperatures dropped below zero. We had three-foot snowdrifts from the north. The cover we built for our new trailers collapsed with the weight of the snow and totaled our brand-new trailer/camper. I was heartbroken. My dreams of camping with the boys were dashed in a moment, along with the hopes of traveling with my husband and taking a motorcycle ride together. I felt like God was saying, "You don't need that now. You need to get these renovations done." It made sense since we had learned a lot about what changes we wanted to make on the house and what upgrades needed to be done. We needed to build a shop. Later, it seemed that all of 2021 involved some renovation and building.

I prayed daily for the right people to come alongside to help with Mitchell. My prayers were answered shortly afterward when Arrie, a yoga therapist, arrived. He overflowed with empathy and was exactly what we needed in Mitchell's life. He committed to coming to the Ranch three days a week, and as I write this book, he is still here, making a difference in our lives. More people were crossing our path, great people who loved Mitchell and let him be part of the work they were doing. He was living in his cabin more and less on our couch, and I was joyful about where we were. However, the numbers from the labs we closely monitored for Mitchell were not improving. They were worse.

In March, God delivered another *angel* to us, Dr. Smith. I chatted on the phone with him for an hour. What doctor today will do that? I knew something was different about this doctor. I could feel it in my soul. Hope was returning. I had no idea if we would find anything new or if he was the one who might lead me to someone else with the answer, but I was living on faith and prayer. I sat still and gave thanks to God and felt great comfort in the security of His peace.

After speaking with me, Dr. Smith came to see Mitchell at our home and met with him in his cabin, which was a step forward for me as I usually had to be present. This time it was just Mitchell and him without interruptions. Afterward, they came walking up to my house with huge smiles. Dr. Smith told Mitchell, "You are in there, and we are going to get you out!" There was a massive smile on my son's face, and I could tell a sense of peace and hope came over him. I thought he was going to cry. I was! I fell to my knees in the grass with a great sense that we were going to win. Mitchell would get his life back! All my fighting would be worth it!

I called my nurse friend Ami from church, and she came to draw blood again. This time Dr. Smith had a new test he was running. It was innovative. We hoped to determine what was happening in Mitchell's brain to cause the drops we had been observing and, God-willing, determine what to do to stop them.

A few short weeks later, Dr. Smith brought Mitchell's test results. We sit down. He opens his laptop and begins to give me the biochemistry. Because I am so familiar with its science, I wanted to understand the chain of events he was uncovering. For the past 15 years, I have thought in terms of chemical equations and functions.

Dr. Smith knew this, so he began to dive deep into the data, explaining what he found. The more he talked, the tighter my chest got, the harder it was for me to breathe. The missing links were showing up, the absent molecules. As he neared the end of his explanation, THERE IT WAS!! Significant red indicators on the screen.

Inside your brain is something called the blood-brain barrier, and Mitchell's had holes in his causing a viral leak into his brain, causing his brain to be in a critical autoimmune state. A condition that is referred to as "brain on fire." Mitchell's neurons were shorting out everywhere. His own body's immune system was attacking his brain and creating blocks on any attempts for him to process information, especially from the outside world. Dr. Smith later explained that he believed the multiple undiagnosed concussions weakened his blood-brain barrier and that Mitchell's drug use further complicated the issue. Now I am a bawling crying mess, and I can hardly breathe. We found what needs to be fixed, and, we can fix it!

Dr. Smith called Mitchell and Jacob over to tell them what he had discovered. He explained, "Mitchell, you have holes in part of your brain that allowed a virus to infect your brain. The virus attacked your brain, causing your psychoses, body function degeneration, confusion, hallucinations, hearing voices, and inability to speak. Everything is because of the virus." Mitchell is welling up with tears, and I am about to pass out from holding my breath. Then Dr. Smith spoke what we had longed to hear. "AND WE CAN FIX IT."

I remember Mitchell saying the words, "I not a bad kid. I not a bad kid." Dr. Smith hugged him and told him, "No, sir. Mitchell Lee Smith is an amazing kid. And we are going to close these holes and get this virus out of you." I was so overwhelmed. I could not handle it anymore. I walked away crying so hard I could not see. I put on my headphones and got on my riding lawn mower, and took some time to gather all this unfathomable information into my heart. It's hard to put to words the relief I felt. I prayed and praised the Lord excessively. There is HOPE!! Wild hope! Powerful hope! Every day

I am sustained by prayer, faith, and hope. This day, God was squeezing me tight, saying, "Let's go! We're going to fix this." The God Gap was the place where I found the answer and the person who could fix the problem. Only God! Only God can guide us on our journey. Thank God for His helper the Holy Spirit.

In April, we doubled down on systemic nutrients, added a few other vital nutritional molecules, and used a specially formulated peptide nasal spray that went directly to Mitchell's brain to rebuild the blood-brain barrier. Within forty-eight hours, Mitchell was more precise and aware. We could see the change visibly. His pace increased, and he started saying more words in a timely fashion. We had a new protocol of nutritional medicine to keep his body systemically healthy and robust, necessary to fight this virus and speed healing to close the holes and stop the brain leak. I plan to share all the protocols in my next book in greater detail. We hit the mark, revealing the cause with the proper test regarding Mitchell.

By May, Mitchell is waking up! We see changes in his focus, movement, and timing function. Praise God! It is time to ramp up movement and lifestyle medicine to take advantage of this healing time to grow and connect as many neuro pathways as possible. We are still not sure how much retraining will be necessary, but Mitchell's function is increasing throughout June, July, and August, and his lab numbers are rising. We live one day at a time and praise God for each small step toward healing.

Support personnel abounded, for which we are truly grateful. We brought in a personal trainer, Mark, a counselor skilled in hypnosis, to get Mitchell moving. TJ Martinez, an occupational martial

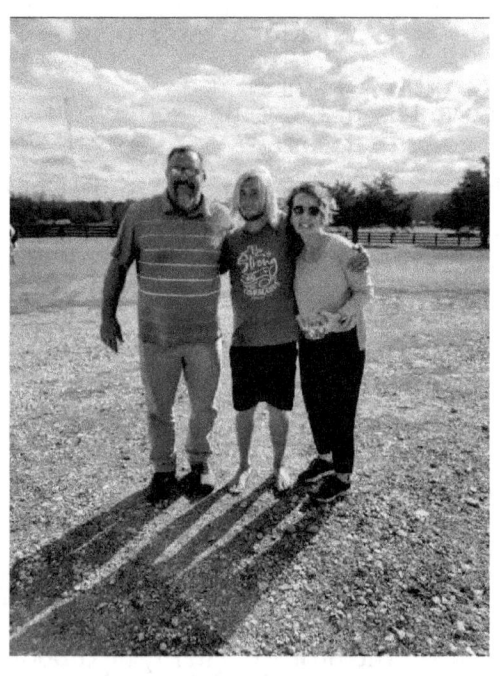

artist, was added to teach Mitchell Taekwondo. My massage therapist Valerie Simpson came to the Ranch to massage Mitchell. She also introduced us to Mitchie and Michael, who were *angels*.

These two miraculous humans, a counselor, and a business owner, are Bible study teachers. They host a Bible Study Fellowship for college-aged students who are uniquely "outside the box." They welcomed Mitchell into their Tuesday fellowship, bringing a new dynamic to his interaction and growth.

As each person came, it brought me a new level of surrender, requiring me to let go and allow others to serve us without any expectations of something from us in return. It was a difficult concept for me to grasp because I had always been the giver. Surprisingly, receiving from them required something unexpected from me—courage. It's hard to put it into words, but trusting others to do what was right and best is not an easy thing to do when you've been fighting for every little victory for years. I was required though, by the events as they unfolded, to let others love on us so unconditionally. Initially, I was so uncomfortable in my own skin. I wanted to say, do it this way, say it that way, but the Holy Spirit whispered, "Be still. Let God do the work." In a world where kindness is seldom seen without an ulterior motive, it took every ounce of courage within me to "Let go, and let God."

In September, Dr. Smith ordered more labs to check Mitchell's numbers. We learned in October of 2021 that Dr. Smith's protocol was successful. The holes in Mitchell's brain were CLOSED! A tremendous victory for Mitchell and EVERYONE who had worked with us over the years! Mitchell's brain is no longer leaking, and we are on the right path to destroy the virus that still plagues him. Lifestyle medicine is in full force. Our battle will be over when Mitchell can interweave nutrition, movement, and lifestyle protocols on his own. We are in the home stretch now; the finish line is within our reach.

Autumn was nearing an end. For the first time in six years, Mitchell knew what day it was. He sat at the table with us at Thanksgiving and Christmas without fear controlling his every interaction and thought. On Christmas morning, he opened his presents, inspecting them like a child, a sight that filled me with inexpressible joy. My son was happy. Gratitude flooded my soul. I was so grateful I discovered the God Gap. Where would we be right now if I had not surrendered to the still small voice of my God? His mercy consumed us and changed my focus—something I don't take for granted. I want every parent with a child suffering from some form of ABI to enter that God Gap with me where hope finally abounds and answers come.

Jacob, Arrie, and I sat down with Mitchell for the first time to discuss goals we could set for him. We all agreed that Mitchell would talk, communicating his feelings, desires, and thoughts in 2022. Expressing emotions in words can be a challenge for all of us, but we knew Mitchell wanted to speak. As we discussed his goals, Mitchell agreed, saying clearly, and meaningfully, "I want to talk."

Even now, though I am telling his story, I can see him one day sharing it himself. He has taught me many things over these years of heartbreak, challenge, and determination to find the answers I'd been searching for since I first started horse therapy for kids with behavioral issues. He's taught me how to have patience and empathy, how to be brave and love unconditionally at a deeper level than I could ever imagine. Mitchell's journey also revealed the reality of my heart, which is singly the most painful part of his story, yet the most liberating of it all. Through each step, I found Christ in a way that broke my heart as I came face-to-face with Him. The life lessons have been profound but worth revisiting, though. I never want to forget one of them as we journey through the rest of our lives, learning and growing in the God Gap.

— Chapter 10 —

LESSONS I LEARNED ALONG THE WAY

As I endeavor to bring this book to a close, I want to leave you with an action plan for your children and family who may also be struggling with an ABI or other mental "giants" by diagnosis or label. I also want to share my painful yet necessary life lessons for your growth and success.

Friend, I know you have struggled in your life; we all do. However, there are answers to every challenge. Journeying through them requires determination and persistence, as well as an openness to allow what is unseen and unknown to come into your life. God, Who the whole of creation exists within, has every answer, a plan for you to follow, and victory out ahead. You must decide to let Him take control, listen intently, and do what He inspires you to do. He has a beautiful way of allowing us to get to the end of ourselves, position us to receive, even open our ears and eyes to hear and see. All we have to do is acknowledge Him and ask, which was the greatest lesson I learned. It proved to be the exact part of our journey that God miraculously prepared with everything and everyone we would need along the way. While the path we walked out was heart-wrenching, the victories and relationships we formed were priceless.

One thing is for sure, walking through a challenge like ours is a step-by-step process. I've thought a lot about those steps and I think they may help you through your challenges too. Let me take a moment to share them with you, in hopes they will make your journey much easier than mine.

THINK OUTSIDE THE BOX

First, think outside the box. You've probably heard the old saying, "There's more than one way to skin a cat." It means that there are more ways to look at, analyze, and perceive how to approach a situation. Like there is more than one route to get to most locations. The same is true regarding wellness matters. And, we, even science, still have a lot to learn, which is why I love to research. We discover new things, approaches, responses, and protocols from one generation to the next. Be willing to consider alternatives and do your best to learn and discover them.

NEVER TAKE NO AS THE FINAL ANSWER

Next, never take "No" as the final answer. No doesn't mean never. It means not yet, or there's another way. Keep searching, keep inquiring, pray, ask God to release the wisdom needed. Ask Him to bring the people with the answers. Ask Him, but never stop with a "No." Let that answer spur you on to inquire more. Pay attention to the people around you; some are Divinely placed.

Don't miss them.

LEAVE NO STONE UNTURNED

If you have a thought or an idea, find the expert in the field or area of your concern. People, even experts, are more willing to help than you can imagine today. Empathetic people do exist. They need to hear from you and to hear your situation.

INVITE GOD INTO EVERY SITUATION

I've learned that God is a gentleman. He gave us free will, which means we get to choose. He wants to be involved in our lives but waits for us to open the door to Him. I stumbled into the God Gap; I want you to march boldly into the *God Gap* right now. It all begins with one plea, "Help me!" Do that today, even if you don't have a dire situation like mine. Invite Him in.

PRAY, PRAY, PRAY

Start talking to God. That's what prayer is, talking to God. Tell Him everything, even though He already knows it all. He likes having a relationship with us in conversation. I'm thinking here of a verse in James' Book that reads, "We have not because we ask not..." In other words, we don't have what we need because we did not ask God for it. We have to pray and ask God for what we need and desire.

TRUST, TRUST, TRUST

After you pray, believe. Have faith in God. Trust Him. His plans for you and your loved one are good. He has a future filled with hope for you. Trusting God can be difficult to settle into from time to time. We often pray and grow weary when we think God takes too long to answer. What is too long? I've learned that God's timing is perfect. Trust that He is at work in your situation even when you cannot see it. Never lose hope. It is an earnest expectation of future good. Trust is expectation. Keep looking for, watching, and waiting for the fulfillment of what you have asked God to do.

STAY THE COURSE

Simply put, never give up. Never fall short of victory. The process can be grueling, but maintain a mindset of victory. Don't let fear, anxiety, doubt, or worry become more significant than your determination to see victory, which will look different for each situation. Victory may be one tiny step or word spoken. Celebrate every victory, no matter how small, then press on for the next one until you finish!

LESSONS I'VE LEARNED

Life lessons can be hard, but when we embrace the fact that we are imperfect people who need to learn and grow, we become sensitive to what we need to recognize in every challenge that God means for our blessing and growth. Here are some of the most profound life lessons I learned through Mitchell's injury and recovery process.

STOP HIDING & TELL THE TRUTH

Recognizing I was hiding the truth hurt me deeply. I didn't want to admit that I was not the best mother to Mitchell. I put my work before him, my husband, and my marriage. I was driven to do something good for others but at the sacrifice of my family. And I paid a considerable price for it. I lost the things I loved the most, Morning Glory Ranch, staff, families, clients, etc. I'd built what others might have considered an empire, but at the cost of the people, that should have mattered most. Then when everything crumbled, I had to take a hard look in the mirror. God's grace and mercy were available at every turn when what I deserved from man's perspective was everything I was experiencing; shame, remorse, and feelings of the worst guilt for it all.

Acknowledging the truth and telling it to others is the most freeing thing you can ever do for yourself. When you hide, you can't get the help that God has for you, whether from Him or others. It makes me think of Jesus who said, "If my words abide in you, you are My disciples, you will know the truth, and the truth will make you free." While the truth I'm talking about here was the facts about myself and my situation, it still applies. When we tell the truth, we open the door to help. We untie God's hands and loose the healing restoration needed in our hearts.

LET GO

Now I know that surrender is a most beautiful word. When I was running hard and fast before and after Mitchell's brain injury, I have to admit surrender was not part of my vocabulary or lifestyle. However, the moment I let go of everything and said, "God help!" He took over, and I recognized His fingerprints immediately. He was all over the legal help we received, the connections to the people we made, and the progress Mitchell experienced. I'd found the God Gap, and the doorway to it was complete surrender.

I don't ever want to live again outside of surrender. I encourage you to stop resisting God. Let go and let Him take over. The outcome will be more magnificent than you can imagine today.

BE GRATEFUL & LOVE UNCONDITIONALLY

The power twins to a beautiful life are gratitude and love. No matter the circumstances, how grave they may be, always exude a heart of gratitude and love. Every person, every opportunity has a heaven-sent lining if we pay attention. If you start expecting and looking for miracles, you will see them, even if it is a cool breeze or an unexpected call from a friend checking to see how you are or telling you they are praying for you.

DEVELOP EMPATHY FOR OTHERS

One of the big things I realized was that I didn't fully comprehend empathy. I'd served so many families in emotional distress, but I couldn't wholly relate until I knew how they felt and what they were going through. I'm not talking about having compassion or sympathy here either; there's a difference. Compassionate people are willing to relieve the suffering of others, sympathetic people understand what others are going through, but empathetic people feel what others are feeling.

It's profound! When you see others suffering and painstakingly trying to help their loved ones do even the simplest things in life, they are emotionally and often physically drained. They need help, and they need people who can feel what they are feeling.

CLOSING

As I close, I want you to know that you are not alone. There are people who will come alongside to help you. They want to help you;

they just haven't met you yet. Making connections is the most vital thing you can do right now. Find a support group of individuals going through the same thing you are. Get involved with them, share with them, let them help you.

And, get yourself into the God Gap immediately. I left one piece of the puzzle for now, and it's the essential piece. Jesus! There's one way to God, and it's through faith in Jesus. We're imperfect; He is not. He made a way for us; we only need to repent, believe, and let Him be the Lord of our lives. You need Him in your corner. You also need the peace He gives and the healing He brings.

I don't want to think about what life might look like for Mitchell, David, and me right now if I hadn't found the God Gap, recommitted my life to Jesus, and followed His every leading. I'm confident it would not be what it is today.

One last sweet Mitchell miracle, his dad came to see him on Christmas day. He doesn't visit often. The last time they were together was over a year ago when Mitchell returned from Utah. The joy Mitchell had this time was indescribable. I could see in

Mitchell's eyes that he felt content and full of peace, almost serene. The atmosphere was filled with love, and this momma's heart was bursting again with gratitude for God Who orchestrated that moment for Mitchell and blessed me with an opportunity to witness it all.

There's only one thing left to say to you again. It bears repeating. Get in the God Gap. Get in and stay. Learn to live from that place, and your life will never be the same again.

ABOUT THE AUTHOR

Kim Russell, M.Ed. is internationally recognized in functional behavior nutrition research for moms with children of acquired brain injuries (ABIs).

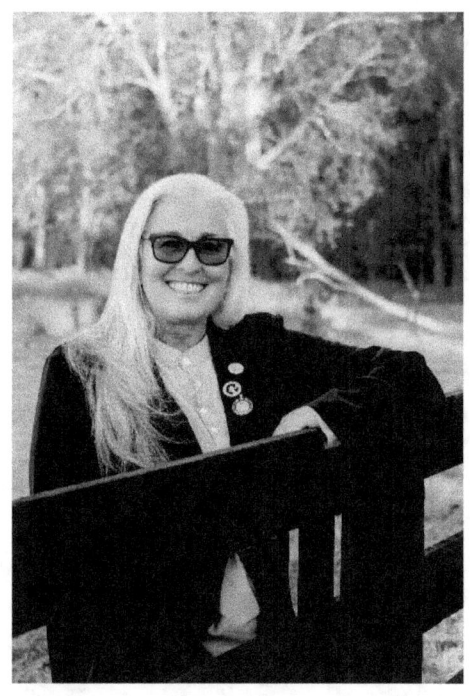

She is the Founder of the Morning Glory Ranch, now a foundation for ABI research and solutions. Kim completed her first piece of research on cellular carotenoid anti-oxidant, absorption, and functional behavior in 2016 through the Morning Glory Ranch Equine Therapy research program serving over 2000 children with Autism and other ABIs.

She is a dedicated mom to her son, Mitchell, who himself acquired a brain injury at age 19. She is also dedicated to her husband, David, and her older children, Michael and Kaydee.

Kim has presented her research and results worldwide regarding the challenges of the children she has served through her foundation. Her organization provides the support they need, especially in basic cellular nutrition absorption.

Kim believes that Jesus is our healer. God loved us so much that He gave His only begotten Son so that we could have life. God's love covers us all, and His love grows in the God Gap, where miracles beyond science abound.

All proceeds of this and subsequent books will fund innovative solutions for ABI. Use this code at checkout:

MorningGloryRanch

Contact Information:

Kim Russell, M.Ed.

Email: mgloryranch@gmail.com

Website: morninggloryranch.net

Facebook Page: The Best of Morning Glory Ranch

Photo Credit

Grace Photography by Jill Ingram Sellers

gracephotographybyjill@gmail.com